RAISING HEALTHY CHILDREN

Health and Nutrition Information, Recipes, and Resources

Nancy Addison

Nancy Alisa Gibbons Addison
www.OrganicHealthyLifestyle.com
www.NancyAddison.com

ISBN-10: 0-9961085-0-5
ISBN-13: 978-0-9961085-0-8
Library of Congress number 2014907691

Limits of Liability and Disclaimer of Warranty

The author and publisher shall not be liable for your misuse of this material. This book is strictly for informational and educational purposes. Nancy Gibbons Addison offers information and opinions, not a substitute for professional medical prevention, diagnosis or treatment. Please consult with your physician, pharmacist, or healthcare provider before taking any home remedies or supplements, or following any treatment suggested by Nancy Gibbons Addison, or by anyone listed in the books, articles, or other information contained here. Only your healthcare provider, personal physician, or pharmacist can provide you with advice on what is safe and effective for your unique needs or diagnose your particular medical history.

Warning – Disclaimer

The purpose of this book is to educate and entertain. The author and publisher do not guarantee that anyone following these techniques, suggestions, tips, ideas, or strategies will become successful. The author and/or publisher shall have neither liability nor responsibility to anyone with respect to any loss or damage caused, or alleged to be caused, directly or indirectly by the information contained in this book.

Medical Disclaimer: Information provided in this book is for informational purposes only. The information is a result of years of practice and experience by Nancy Addison CHC, AADP. However, this information is NOT intended as a substitute for the advice provided by your physician or other healthcare professional. Information provided in this book and the use of any products or services related to this book by you *does not* create a counselor-client relationship between you and Nancy Addison, CHC, AADP.

Do not use the information provided in this book for diagnosing or treating a health problem or disease, or prescribing medication or other treatment. Always speak with your physician or other healthcare professional before taking any medication or nutritional, herbal, or homeopathic supplement, or using any treatment for a health problem. If you have or suspect that you have a medical problem, contact your healthcare provider promptly. Do not disregard professional medical advice or delay in seeking professional advice because of something you have read in this book.

Full Disclosure: If you purchase anything I recommend in this or any of my communications, it's possible I'll receive some kind of affiliate compensation. I only recommend people and programs I believe in deeply, and feel you will get enormous value from. However, if you ever have an issue with something I recommend, please let me know and share your thoughts.

"Nancy Addison's book is a comprehensive guidebook to creating long-term, sustainable, and life-enhancing strategies for raising healthier children through nutrition. In this book, she inspires, motivates, and teaches easy-to-implement suggestions as well as offers incredible insight into health and wellness. Nancy also has delicious recipes for the whole family. This book gives a parent the power of healthy choices."

—Gary L. Massad, MD, FACOM, FAASM, FAC, LM.
Past attending physician to the 1984 and 1996 Olympic Games, attending physician to United States Cycling Federation, USTAA, and USMAA

Being a mother, raising my children in the happiest and healthiest way possible was my most important and cherished job. I wouldn't trade it for anything in the world. Don't let the little moments escape. Capture them in your heart and hold onto them forever. For it is the little unexpected moments that send pure joy into your soul and make life worth living.

—Nancy Addison

DEDICATION AND ACKNOWLEDGMENTS

First and foremost, I thank God for the constant love, support, inspiration, knowledge, experiences, and energy that it took to put this book together. May God bless this book and all who read it.

Heartfelt thanks and dedication to my children, ***Amanda Gibbons Addison*** and ***Frederick Gibbons Addison***. It was you who provided the inspiration for writing this book, to share our special recipes and tips with others. You are the loves of my life and my biggest fans, and I am yours. It has been my biggest joy in the world to be your mother. You two have hung in there with me through thick and thin as my foundation and support while I experimented with food and life in all its venues. As my original taste-testers, you helped me prepare, develop, refine, and taste-test all of my new ideas all of your lives. I am so very blessed to call myself your mother. My heart overflows with love for you. Thank you for a lifetime of your unwavering support and love.

Thanks to my wonderful parents, Junia and Patrick. You raised and took care of five children with devotion and love. You cooked every day the best food you knew how to make. You've tried to help us with all the decisions we have had to make. You were there for every single occasion you could possibly attend, which was just about all of them! You set a strong example for us to learn from. Thank you for everything.

Thank you to my sister Jane, her husband David, their child Claire and her husband Stefan, and their children Audrey and Reid. Thank you to my sister Liz, her husband Layne, and their children: Jack and his wife Amber, and their children Annie and Ford; Clayton and his wife Lynsie, and their child Scout. Thanks to my brother Patrick and his son

Ryan; to my sister Mary, her husband Rusty, and their children, Carter, Katie, and Rebecca. Your love and support for my children and me has been a godsend. You enrich my life every day. I'm so fortunate to be a part of this family.

Thank you to my precious daughter-in-law Edy and her wonderful parents Chip and Cynthia Jones. I am honored with your love, generosity, encouragement, friendship, and support. I love your family, and I am thrilled to share my son with you.

An enormous thank you to Dr. Gary Massad for his consistent faith, support, and encouragement. I will be forever grateful.

To all of the wonderful friends and neighbors from my life who have honored me with their friendship, never-ending patience, cheerful words of encouragement, and constant support, I thank you all for making my life so much brighter. Bless you all.

Thank you to Joshua Rosenthal and Institute of Integrative Nutrition; Carole Maureen Friesen and Hermann Müller with Body Mind Communications of psychosomatic therapy; T. Colin Campbell and your classes with Cornell University on the plant-based diet; Natural Gourmet Institute for Food and Health; Alissa Cohen; Australasian College of Health and Science; Tree of Life; National Speakers Association and all the friends I've made there. I have loved this journey with you.

Thank you to all of my friends and associates at Allie Beth Allman and Associates for your kindness, generosity, and encouragement. Also thanks to all of my friends from Highland Park for your encouragement, faith, and friendship through the years.

Thank you to my ex-husband, Rick, the father of my children, for sharing with me our two wonderful children.

My Appreciation for Contributors to This Book

A special thank you to Sharyn Wynters for contributing the Foreword to this book. I am deeply honored by your contribution and grateful for your time, effort, faith, generosity, and support. It has been a real pleasure knowing you and sharing our passions for healthier living.

My thanks to Michael W. Hall, DC, FIACN, for contributing a chapter on chiropractic care. I am extremely honored you took the time and energy to do so. Your special gift of sharing preventative and natural healing methods with the world is exceptional. It has been a pleasure knowing you and your amazing wife and fabulous family. You have been so generous in so many ways. Please accept my heartfelt thanks.

A special thank you to Chef Terry French for his scrumptious recipe and contribution about raising his children. It has been a joy getting to know such a generous, kind, and talented chef and father. I admire you for your hard work to make the world a place where no child will ever be hungry.

A deep, heartfelt thank you to my thoughtful, delightful, and generous friend Linda Gray for her kind contribution of delicious, healthy recipes! You have been so gracious to take the time and energy to contribute your special family recipes, and I'm incredibly blessed to have you in my life.

A special thank you to Dr. Cynthia Champion-Olson for your incredible thoughtfulness, generosity of spirit, encouragement, expertise, and input. I greatly appreciate your time and effort as well as your advice and contributions to my knowledge. I am blessed to know you and have you in my life.

To my dear, sweet sisters Liz Newman and Mary Katherine Dean, my wonderful mother Junia, my fantastic daughter Amanda, my amazing son Gibbons, Gibbons's wife Edy, and my dear and talented friends Maryann De Leo, Suzie Humphreys, and Leslee Carr

Feiwus for contributing recipes. I am honored to have them appear in this book.

Thank you to my dear friend Lisa Endicott of Lisa Endicott PR and staff for all you have done for me with skill, expertise, thoughtfulness, and kind consideration. You have been there with me throughout all my journeys. You've enriched my life, and it has been a delight to work with you.

A special thank you to Susan Doyle, Cindy Williams, Deanna Sweet, Adele Good, Stephanie Askew, Mark Pharo, Charlotte Ammerman, Kirk Dooley, Michael Reisman, Dr. Bill Osmunson, DDS, Nick Sakulenzki, Kelley Willis, Dr. Sandra Bontemps, DC, Priscilla Miller, Janneth Whitworth , Kytka Hilmar-Jezek, Julianne Parker, Eve Baughman Yung, Suann Davis, Dr. Therese Rowley, Kimberly Wechsler, Alan Rodriguez, Earl Rector, Susan Staples, Susan Williams, Karis Adams, Trish Aldredge, Kurt Boxdorfer, Dr. Anitra Thorhaug, Julie Goss, Judd Walker, Lori Markman, Mary Monttein Alonso, Debbie Russell, Nancy Miller, Mary Jo Rausch, Kathleen Hayden, Nancy Miller, Cindy Williams, Richard Kemp, Andrea and Randy Harrah, Harrison Evans, Chris Koustoubardis, Prudie and Rick Koeninger, Ralph Kubitzki, Marilyn Flemming, Rhett Stein, Donza Doss, Candace Stone, Becky Crow Nolan, Jacqueline Cornaby, Vanessa Mickan, Orvel Ray Wilson, Gina Carr, Tim Durkin, Dave Lieber, Bev Garvin, Jimmy Wynne and so many friends who have helped me in more ways than I can list.

Thank you to my Health Nuts Group: Sheila Fitzgerald, Dr. Mary Warren, Dr. Elizabeth Naylor, Dean Vanderslice and Denise Ringer. It has been a fun and interesting journey with you.

Thanks to all of my dear friends at the National Speakers Association and the north Texas chapter for all your help, support, kindness, and generosity. I am very grateful for you. A warm thank you to Dr. Jan Goss for believing in me. Thank you for your support and continued encouragement.

Thank you, Matthew Howard, for helping me finalize this book with design support, copyediting, and proofreading. Thank you, Gwyn Snider of GKS Creative, for helping me with cover and interior design.

An enormous thank you to Kytka Hilmar-Jezek who has been an angel in so many things concerning this book that I can't even count them. Thank you, Kytka, for making my Kindle version and so much more!

Thanks to my fabulous photographer Elizabeth Glover for my author's photo in this book. An additional thank you to Barbara McNichol, my amazingly incredible editor who helped me get it all together. You went way beyond the call of duty! I am grateful for all of your outstanding hard work and dedication to this project. It has been an honor to work with you.

I am grateful for all of you. Bless you all. Please accept my deepest, heartfelt thanks.

CONTENTS

FOREWORD

by Sharyn Wynters

Years ago while pursuing a career in acting, I developed severe health problems that the medical profession could not treat successfully. My life took a unique turn as I looked to complementary and alternative medicine. While researching, I discovered the steady, subtle undermining of our health in conjunction with the advent of pesticides, processed foods, unnatural electromagnetic fields, and thousands of chemicals that had not existed on the planet before. These factors and more have contributed to an increasingly toxic environment.

As our exposure increases, the incidence of cancer, immune deficiency, heart disease, diabetes, and other chronic ailments are reaching epidemic proportions. Yet, it is our children who will pay the ultimate price. More than ever, children suffer from headaches, nervous disorders, skin conditions, respiratory problems, and other symptoms that, until now, have been associated with age. They suffer from learning disabilities and behavioral problems that were unheard of years ago.

Anyone with an inquiring mind must ask the question, "Why?"

The growing number of chemicals and other toxins in our environment are bad enough for adults, but for our children, they can be devastating. Children, whose brains, organs, and systems are still developing up to the age of 21, tend to draw toxins into their developing bodies. Modern toxins in all their forms are one of the biggest deterrents to the health and happiness of our children. But it doesn't have to be that way.

My personal health challenges led me to make changes in my lifestyle. As I eliminated processed and pesticide-ridden foods, as I got rid of toxic cleaners and personal care products with less-than-healthy ingredients, and as I focused on healthy, supportive relationships, my health returned. My life focus shifted, and I became a naturopath to show others how to reclaim their health.

Why should you have to *reclaim* your health?

If you are taught from childhood the importance of a healthy, nontoxic lifestyle, your chances of living a long and healthy life are magnified many times. The process must begin when you are young. If my mother had understood the principles of *Raising Healthy Children*, I might never have experienced my own life-threatening health issues.

Raising Healthy Children is a complete guide for parents interested in giving their children a fair start in life. Nancy Addison has gathered all the essentials and put them together in a beautifully written masterpiece. It includes everything from healthy options in food (with dozens of fun recipes) to creating the best water and selecting personal care products that will support rather than weaken your child's health. But, one of the most delightful aspects of *Raising Healthy Children* is seeing into another woman's experience.

Many mothers have tried to adopt a healthier lifestyle and environment for their children, only to be sabotaged by family, school, and community. It is not easy to be accused of being a fanatic or of depriving your children of unhealthy "treats" during childhood. Nancy shares her struggles and her successes as she forged ahead, committed to giving her daughter and son the very best. In this book, she shares her experiences teaching the principles of healthy food preparation from gardening to table garnish.

As you read *Raising Healthy Children,* you will gain wonderful insights into raising children with love. You will catch a glimpse of how a mother's whole heart can go into the experience. Best of all, you will know you can do it, too!

As a naturopath, much of what I do is educating those who come to me for assistance. *Raising Healthy Children* is a foundational work for providing both education and the incentive to change. As a free society, we have choices. However, those choices are often made in ignorance without complete or accurate information. The act of choosing is often tainted by those who may not have our best interests at heart. *Raising Healthy Children* brings much-needed awareness and education to the table.

Our children are endowed with a birthright to live in a clean and balanced environment, to eat nutritious food, to fill their lungs with fresh, unpolluted air, and to enjoy the bounty of our divine heritage. *Raising Healthy Children* will guide you in helping your children to realize their birthright. Read it from cover to cover, try the recipes, and adhere to the principles. Fall in love with *Raising Healthy Children.*

Sharyn Wynters is an author and naturopath who advocates whole food nutrition and toxin-free living. Her latest book, The Pure Cure: A Complete Guide to Freeing Your Life From Dangerous Toxins *delves into the dangers of the toxins in our environment and how to avoid them.*

INTRODUCTION

My Life Journey with Food, Health, and Family

I grew up in a family of five children on a half-acre lot with parents who loved to garden, cook, and have regular family meals together. It's no wonder I am now an avid gardener and chef. But that wasn't always true.

As a small child, I helped my parents with the garden. Many a Saturday morning was spent weeding or watching my father plant another fruit tree. My parents invested hours in the kitchen creating gourmet preserves, dishes, and drinks from the bounty of produce they harvested. Our kitchen was definitely the heart of our home. My siblings and I often helped our mother prepare meals. We were also taste testers for yet one more type of mayonnaise, chutney, sandwich, or dish my father or mother invented that day. A love of cooking, working with the earth, and being creative were given high priority in our lives.

Following Directions

My parents dutifully tried to follow the nutritional guidelines our doctors suggested. My mother bought margarine, vegetable shortening, and fortified bread and milk, believing they were important for our health and well-being. My parents were particularly concerned about proper eating, because when I was two I was admitted to the hospital after the doctor gave me an overdose of penicillin. They were told I would die before the next morning. I received several blood transfusions and bone marrow tests. Well, miracles do happen, and I survived. My father told me that was the night he truly embraced God.

As a result of this incident, though, I was left with acute anemia. Being a skinny, anemic child, I developed an extreme taste for sugar and the energy rush it gave me. It wasn't unusual for me to have desserts every chance I got. I loved to make sugar and butter sandwiches on soft white bread for an after-school snack. By the time I was in high school, my doctor told my mother that if I wasn't careful, I would end up with diabetes. My mother dug in and became a strict overseer of everything I put in my mouth. I was given a concerned talk and told exactly what was necessary for me to be healthy. From then on, sweets were kept to a minimum. My mother made high-protein breakfasts, lunches, and dinners for me, which helped me avoid getting diabetes. That's when I became aware that sugar wasn't a good choice, and that diet and health are directly connected.

About this time, artificial sweeteners were coming on the market. My doctor told me they were good for people like me who shouldn't eat "normal" sugar. So diet sodas became a supposedly "healthy" drink of choice for me.

Fascination with Food

College offered a new food adventure. I tried to stick to my mother's healthy guidelines, but at times, peanut M&Ms and fast food won out. During my sophomore year, I lived in London, England. There, I enrolled in classes at Le Cordon Bleu London school of culinary arts and found my element. Food became a fun and delicious adventure. Next, I took Chinese gastronomy courses at the University of London. What better way to learn than cooking gourmet meals for my college class? It was heaven.

After returning to Dallas a few years later, I got married and continued my fascination with food. I wanted to learn everything there was to know about gourmet cuisine. That's when I was driven to find out how to make the best strawberry soufflé in the world. In fact, I became the soufflé queen, also mastering broccoli soufflés, cheese soufflés, and chocolate soufflés.

Then I began volunteering at the Lighthouse for the Blind, working with a group of older individuals who had lost their vision. We were supposed to help them learn the nuances of surviving and thriving. It was particularly hard for some of them who had once made their living using their sight. Because they couldn't go for a run or watch TV, many became extremely depressed or suicidal. As an artist and certified art teacher in Texas, I started a pottery class where these folks could socialize and use their creativity. In the class, I taught them how to make simple pieces of art out of clay. They would tell me they could "see" their art pieces in their mind's eye and even visualize the color they'd paint them. Creating pottery made them happy, which made me incredibly happy, too.

Dealing with Carpal Tunnel Syndrome

Unfortunately, I was overworking my hands and developed carpal tunnel syndrome. It reached a point of excruciating pain just to make a fist or use my hands. Taking a break from teaching pottery, I saw doctors about the pain. They had me wear hand splints and told me I needed cortisone shots. Those painful shots did bring relief for a short while. Then the doctors suggested I have surgery. Rather than agreeing to surgery, I set out to use alternative solutions first. That's when I started to read in earnest about carpal tunnel and natural ways to heal it.

At the same time, I was learning how to make wonderful cappuccinos and lattes. My brother worked at Starbucks and taught me to use one of its great espresso machines. Drinking at least two lattes a day, I started having severe headaches. My doctor asked me how much caffeine I was consuming. It surprised me to realize I had become a caffeine addict. To deal with this addiction, I went cold turkey and gave up all caffeine for about three months—a habit I didn't believe I'd *ever* be able to give up.

After a while, I slowly allowed myself one cup of coffee a day. Now, many years later, I don't drink coffee every day, but I do allow myself to have it occasionally as if it were dessert.

Around that time, I also started studying omega-3 fatty acids. I discovered that when I ate concentrated, nutrient-dense, raw foods daily, and added good oils including omega-3s and evening primrose oil, my hands felt better. How was my diet actually affecting my health? I needed to know!

Motherhood and Weight Gain

The day I found out I was expecting a baby, my husband and I felt thrilled. At the time, I weighed only 100 pounds and suddenly found myself ravenous for food. I couldn't stop eating. My doctor told me my body was trying to make up for my lack of fat and said not to worry about how much I ate. He didn't tell me exactly what to eat, except he suggested foods that contained iron, such as liver, because of my acute anemia.

He also said I had hypoglycemia and had to eat even more, so I ate and ate and ate. When we were blessed with a healthy baby girl, my urge to eat quickly disappeared. I was still overweight, though, and needed to get back to my regular weight. The doctor told me not to worry; the weight would come off as I breastfed our baby. He also said I couldn't get pregnant while I was breastfeeding. Not true. Four months later, I was pregnant again and still overweight. Even though I was ravenous again, I tried not to eat all the time. Again, my doctor told me not to worry. I could eat normally as long as I took my prenatal vitamins. So for the remainder of the pregnancy, I ate voraciously, unable to control the cravings. When I delivered a healthy baby boy, I weighed about 50 pounds more than my average weight. In fact, I was so overweight I actually had three chins!

Determined to lose that weight, I started taking a ballet class two nights a week. I felt self-conscious seeing myself in a ballet studio mirror wearing a leotard made for pregnant women, but I dug in and attended classes faithfully while dreaming of wearing a smaller-sized leotard.

Beyond motivating me, ballet became food for my soul. It strengthened my body's core. Because I'd had two Ceasarean deliveries, my stomach muscles were weak, and my back hurt tremendously. Ballet helped rebuild my stomach muscles and quell my back pain as well as improve my posture.

In addition, being with two babies most of my day, I enjoyed being around adults in a different type of environment. I loved the camaraderie of my classmates, and when I lost myself in the dance and music, the rest of the world totally melted away.

I simply love this art form. Taking ballet was one of the best things I ever did for myself.

Love of Animals

About this time, I read a *LIFE* magazine article about corporate factory farms and the drugs they were giving animals to fatten them faster than ever. The article expanded on the horrific conditions these pigs, birds, and livestock live in. Because of these conditions, they also gave them antibiotics to keep them alive. Years later, I also learned about the environmental destruction and pollution fostered by these types of farms.

I'm an animal lover, and knowing about the cruel treatment of these animals made my heart hurt. So I turned to my husband, an environmental trial lawyer, and told him I could never again participate in purchasing and eating food from these corporations.

My father, who had survived a heart attack when I'd just finished college, developed cancer. I started thinking about my family history of heart disease, cancer, arthritis, and ulcers. I had lost all of my grandparents when they were fairly young.

Sadly, my father died when my son was only one year old. This became a significant turning point for me. Given my family history of heart disease, cancer, and arthritis, *and* being from Texas, I'd always eaten a Western and Southern diet rich in meat and fried foods.

Members of our family had always done everything the doctor said. But after losing my father, I knew there must be a way to better health. That's when I resolved to get healthy, stay healthy, and bring up my children to be as healthy as possible. Besides, I wanted to see my grandchildren grow up and to feel well enough to enjoy being with them!

A New Journey to Health

So picture this: I was overweight with hypoglycemia, acute anemia, and a bad case of acid reflux disease. Then I was diagnosed with scoliosis. To begin my new journey to health, I researched everything I could get my hands on about health, healing, and nutrition.

To be on the safe side, I dutifully had my children's blood and my own checked every year for any kind of deficiency. Many years later, after one of these tests my pediatrician said they were the healthiest children he'd ever seen. Within a couple of years, my weight adjusted to my old normal, my hypoglycemia went away, my acute anemia vanished, and my acid reflux was gone. This made me feel even more enthusiastic about my new nutritional pathway. I knew I was onto something wonderful.

In addition to eating organically, using cloth diapers, and nonchemical household cleaning products, and more, I made my own fresh baby food—now called raw or living food. I also made fresh alternative milks, meals, snacks, and desserts. I was determined that my family would eat the freshest food we could possibly have. More than that, my children wouldn't take in sugar, hormones, antibiotics, or other harmful food additives during the years their organs were forming. And to this, I always added the most important ingredient: my love.

The early years of my healthy lifestyle journey were not without challenges. Where could we buy whole, organic food in Dallas in 1988? Very few groceries offered it. So, I planted an organic garden, joined an organic seed co-op, found select markets with fresh food, and ordered food via mail from organic farms.

When people do something outside the norm, others can feel uncomfortable. In fact, changing my diet and how I was raising my children seemed so threatening to some people, I was called awful names at times. Sometimes, I wasn't invited to certain parties or dinners because other mothers thought I was depriving my children of a "happy, normal childhood." Indeed, some labeled the whole grain, low-sugar snacks I brought to the school as weird or not good.

Still, I forged ahead and tried my best to stick with my new program. I'm not saying I didn't make mistakes, but I learned as I went and made adjustments along the way. Yes, I'm still finding new information all the time. It's a *lifelong* journey.

My children have accompanied me on this journey and learned along with me. They've assisted me as I made food, gardened, and cleaned. We turned our trips to the recycling center across town into adventures filled with joy, music, laughter, and singing. I kept the kids interested by getting their input on what seeds we'd buy and what recipes we'd make. We made it fun!

When I look back, I know this involvement made them feel important, respected, and smart. Being a part of the decisions and processes also motivated them to try and enjoy the foods as well as all the activities.

Healthy Children, Healthy Adults

Today, my children Gibbons and Amanda have graduated from college after somehow surviving their out-of-the-ordinary childhood. They grow herbs, cook whole grain, eat healthy meals, get plenty of exercise, and realize they are much healthier than many others. They even give advice about whole foods to their friends.

Today, several decades after I embarked on this journey, I see increasing numbers of people sick with cancer, diabetes, heart disease, weight problems, and more. Thankfully, my children and I feel well and experience good health. And we're not perceived as out of the ordinary. A broader range of people than ever realize eating a healthful diet isn't as weird as they'd thought. Frankly, I never understood how people couldn't see that what we eat affects every cell in our body. The substances we ingest actually become our blood, our cells, and our tissues. How could it *not* directly affect our health?

When I host a party these days, people love to come and see what kind of food I'm serving. It is quickly gobbled up, complete with praise about being the most delicious food they've ever eaten.

In addition, I've learned so much that I've taken this knowledge and passion to become a certified heath counselor, certified raw food chef, and instructor. I teach others how to grow, prepare, and enjoy fresh, whole, healthy, organic food that can help make them and their families live more vibrant lives. That's why I'm excited to share this information with you in *Raising Healthy Children.*

Welcome to my party!

I embraced this journey of health with a full heart. I know I made mistakes along the way, but I learned from them and tried to do better as I went along.

CHAPTER 1

Lifestyle Aspects of Raising Healthy Children

When I was first married, I taught art at a school for children with learning differences. Some had severe emotional problems and couldn't attend mainstream schools. I had the most severely affected students in my homeroom class. For instance, one boy was obsessed with guillotines, blood, and death. He had been asked to leave more than five schools, and we were his last chance.

While we ate our lunches in my homeroom, I learned what the kids were eating and what kind of home lives they had. I looked at what they'd brought for lunch. We'd talk about the food they ate at home. Many of them ate marshmallows, chips, Twinkies, or salty and sugary fast foods for their snacks or even their main meals. Some made their own lunches of white bread and packaged snack foods. I rarely saw fresh vegetables, whole grain breads, or fresh fruit. In many cases, both of their parents worked and felt they needed to rely on fast food, because they didn't believe they had enough time to prepare healthier meals with fresh food. At the time, many people believed—and many still believe—fast food is reasonably healthy and convenient in their busy lives.

Art reflects society and what is happening at the time. That is why it is so highly valued.

I taught all grade levels of art, drama, and homemaking at a small school of grades 1 to 12. Observing my students taught me a lot, especially when it came to my homemaking class. It was actually a cooking and nutrition class with no guidelines, so I made them up as I went along. We discussed nutrition and vitamins. I taught them how to bake potatoes, even making our own fresh butter to put on them. I also taught them how to steam fresh broccoli and green beans, and how to make a whole fruit-and-nut dessert. They *loved* it. This might have been because they got to eat in class, but they also became empowered by their new knowledge.

Most of these students were on the drug Ritalin. In my opinion, the best thing for children in general—and especially those who have trouble sitting still—is to take them out before every class and let them run around the block. It's amazing what a little exercise, fresh air, and sunshine will do for a child who's expected to sit for hours and concentrate. It did wonders for me, too.

If we consistently do this every hour or two and give the children healthy food, they may not need all of those drugs after all.

Unconditional Love

I also found that many of these children received little to no consistent attention and love from their parents. Maybe both parents worked or the child had only one parent. For the most part, the children rarely experienced one-on-one time with a parent. They'd often go home and stay alone for hours. After a dinner of processed or fast food, they had bathtime and bedtime with a little TV time thrown in. Many of these parents were unaware of a child's need to have eye contact and direct conversation about life without a TV blaring in the background.

I'm not saying the parents weren't working hard to support the family they loved or weren't extremely tired when they got home. I know most of the parents thought they were doing the best they could at the time. I'm only saying that the lack of personal parental attention was taking its toll on these children. What children want most is to have their parents' eyes light up at the sight of them.

> *It is amazing what individual attention and love will do for a child. Unconditional love is the most crucial. It's love that doesn't have to be earned in any way, shape, or form. Just love because of being oneself.*

If we don't receive that unconditional love as a child, then we spend the rest of our lives trying to get it—often in sad ways. Some look for it in gangs or groups of every kind which often involve initiations of tattoos, alcohol, or drugs. Finding unconditional love is a basic need for all living beings.

Mixed Messages

There seems to be a mixed message in giving children drugs for all kinds of ailments. On one hand, adults are telling children, "Do not take drugs." Then, on the other hand, they are saying, "Take these drugs." What is the real message we're giving children? Why is one drug illegal and one not? What is the difference?

I feel this subconsciously tells children that (1) "There is something wrong with you," and (2) "Drugs are okay for solving your problems. Drugs are a quick fix." Are these the messages we want to give our children?

Recently, I learned about a school system in Wisconsin that had a terrible behavior problem to the point of having to hire security guards. The students' scholastic scores were extremely low, and the administrators had trouble hiring teachers to work there. So, they tried an experiment. They initiated a five-year program of having only healthy food in their schools. Would offering only nutritious food make a real difference in the student's behavior, learning, and health?

Here's a statement from this case study:

> In 1997, Greg Bretthauer was offered the job of dean of students at one of the Wisconsin schools. What he saw were teens who were "rude, obnoxious, and ill mannered," and he turned the job down. Because the school had so many problems with discipline and weapons violations, a police officer was recruited to be on the staff.
>
> Today Greg is the dean of students in an atmosphere that is vastly different from what he saw in 1997. Each year, principals are required to file a report with the state of Wisconsin, detailing the number of students who have dropped out, been expelled, been found using drugs or carrying weapons, or committed suicide. Since the start of the program, the numbers in every category have been zero.[1]

Food Additives and Dyes

I have researched how additives, preservatives, and food color dyes can cause so many health problems as well as emotional and behavioral problems in children. ADHD and hyperactivity can be misdiagnosed when they actually result from additives in foods. [2, 3]

Numerous studies I found on food dyes are quite alarming. For example, "In 2007, a carefully designed, randomized, double-blind, placebo-controlled study published in the journal *The Lancet* concluded that a variety of common food dyes and the preservative sodium benzoate cause some children to become measurably more hyperactive and distractible."[4] This wasn't the first time such a link had been established. In 1994, researchers found that 73 percent of children with ADHD responded favorably to an elimination diet that included removing artificial colors.[5]

Increasingly since the 1960s, more people have come to depend on processed foods that contain colored dyes. Many children's foods such as juices, soft drinks, candy, gelatins, breakfast cereals, baked and snack foods, salad dressings, frozen desserts, and even food you wouldn't normally suspect such as pickles or fresh produce, are coated in dye to make them look more pleasing.

A 68-page report called *Food Dyes: A Rainbow of Risks* by the Center for Science in the Public Interest states this:

> In addition to considerations of organ damage, cancer, birth defects, and allergic reactions, mixtures of dyes (and Yellow 5 tested alone) cause hyperactivity and other behavioral problems in some children. Because of that concern, the British government advised companies to stop using most food dyes by the end of 2009, and the European Union is requiring a warning notice on most dye-containing foods after July 20, 2010.[6]

Many major food manufacturers use natural dyes in European foods while still using the *chemical* dyes in the American foods, because there is still no law in the U.S. banning these food dyes. As the *Food Dyes* report discusses:

> Studies of the nine dyes currently approved by the FDA suggest, if not prove, that most of the dyes cause health problems, including cancer, hypersensitivity, or neurotoxicity (including hyperactivity). . . . The health concerns indicate that most dyes fail the FDA's safety requirement 'that there is convincing evidence . . . that no harm will result from the intended use of the color additive.' Fortunately, numerous natural colorings could be used in place of dyes: beet juice, beta-caramel, carotene, carrot juice, chlorophyll, elderberry juice, grape juice/skin, paprika extract, purple corn, purple sweet potato, red cabbage, and turmeric.[7]

In many ways, we may be able to help our children by cleaning up their diet, teaching them to eat healthier and seeing changes *before* we resort to giving them any kinds of medications. In the long run, we would also be teaching them to live a healthier lifestyle free of drugs and free of being labeled with a disorder or thoughts of something being wrong with them. This could benefit them for life.

A Safe Place to Be Creative

My goal when teaching art and drama was to make the classroom a safe place for my students to be creative. I'd say, "There's no right or wrong with art. It's whatever you want it to be. It's a matter of self-expression." And, in my opinion, everything each student created was a masterpiece. We'd matte their pictures and make them look fantastic, even calling their work modern art if the subjects couldn't quite be recognized. I'd brag about the color, stroke, design, and fluidity. It really didn't matter what I said; all of the students believed I loved everything they did. Before long, they were self-confident enough to design difficult works of art I could truly call masterpieces. I always believed if they created it as a form of self-expression, then who was to say it wasn't a masterpiece?

I persuaded the school to put up strips of corkboard in the hall so I could display the students' art all over the school. I would matte their pictures on beautifully colored paper, an easy and inexpensive way to frame their artwork. It made the children proud to see their art hanging in the hall as if in an art museum while adding color and joy to the atmosphere of the school. Back in 1982, this was a new concept.

I planned different lessons but always encouraged individual creativity, even if it meant allowing a student to draw a guillotine. As mentioned earlier, one of my students had been expelled from multiple schools. Our school was his parents' last hope. The boy had been drawing incredibly morose and scary art and sculptures, including guillotines. I had never met children who had such extreme problems before. This was a new challenge for me.

Still, I encouraged this particular student to make his own art and told him people earn incredibly good income creating sets and costumes for horror movies. I also encouraged him to apply for art school. If he wanted to design costumes, sets, and characters for plays, or even horror movies in Hollywood, he had the potential to make a great living.

"No matter what, you have a bright future," I told him. Opening his mind to these new possibilities made him happier and more confident. From then on, his artwork flowed. He even drew rainbows and, on occasion, other positive subjects. After that, he embraced the major role I gave him in my next play, and he made better grades in his other classes. His entire countenance changed and, at the end of the school year, the teachers nominated him for the outstanding student of the year award. This was one of the happiest moments of my teaching career.

Everyone is a Star!

When I organized one big play each school year, I made sure that many of the children with the worst behavioral problems received some of the biggest and best parts. I'd edit the plays so each student would get a minimum of one line. I even had contests for the design of the program. The students with the fewest lines got to do other jobs such as work on sets, design costumes, manage the lights, work as an understudy, help manage sound, be an usher or announcer, or serve refreshments. This greatly increased their confidence and self-esteem. The plays were a great success, and it made me proud to see the joy students took in their group effort and creative problem solving. I discovered that when you show students you believe in them and trust their judgment, they will rise to the occasion and succeed in ways you could never have imagined. But you have to give them that chance.

I loved teaching school and having the freedom to create programs that worked for the children. It made a huge difference in many of their lives. In my own way, I was an art therapist.

There is nothing that can fill that need for love except love. I am grateful for the love I received. It made me who I am. Yes, I'm always a work in progress. But I am a more stable, self-confident one because of that love.

The school administrators supported me and my ideas. They even had me teach a three-hour seminar at a national dyslexia conference after my first year. What a great honor. The best part? My father took time off work, sat in the back of the room, and was there for me in my big moment.

On a Mission

My teaching experience helped me raise my two children. When they were first born, I ordered a *Teach Your Child to Read* kit, a box containing cards with huge red words and phrases. As they grew, I'd hold up each card and we'd rehearse the words twice a day. We did this faithfully for years. I also labeled things around the house: *drawer, door, window, mirror*. My husband and I always talked to Gibbons and Amanda as if they were older than their years, even explaining things as if they already knew about them.

We would play classical music for them, which supposedly increases one's attention span. Since then, I have learned that music can heal. Masaru Emoto, the Japanese scientist who photographed frozen water molecules, theorized that music can even change the aesthetic quality of water molecules. You'll read more about Emoto's work later in this book. When we listen to music, we access the same part of our brain that we use for math and science. Playing classical and other types of music for my children from their prenatal days forward greatly benefited them.

Like little sponges, my children also soaked up the foreign language lullabies I played. As babies, their tiny brains recorded sight, sound, smell, touch, and taste—a sensory smorgasbord that serves them their whole lives. When I learned that babies take in more in the first year than in the rest of their years put together, I embraced this idea. I also learned that children between the ages of one and six have no filters. They're learning everything as if they are in a hypnotic state, downloading programs and ideas into their brain. This learning can actually become the basis of their self-identity for the rest of their lives.[8]

My children had animals to raise, piles of sand to play in, swings of all kinds, art materials galore, and gardens to grow, explore, and enjoy. What a wonderful, fun time we had together.

To foster self-belief and make their lives rich, vibrant, secure, and loving, I told my children daily they were brilliant, beautiful, and talented. Experts say that whatever parents tell their children about themselves at this young age will be lodged in their subconscious for the rest of their lives.[10] It's incredibly important.

Rosemary for Remembrance

I love plants and the fragrances of flowers and plants. Smell is one of our most powerful senses. I always grew heirloom roses, herbs, vegetables, fruits, and flowers.

In my research, I discovered people who smelled rosemary or peppermint as they took an exam scored as much as 20 percent higher on their tests! I've since learned they do even better if they smell the same scent while studying and then again when taking the test. The scents stimulate the brain and relax the person. They're also good for memory. In recent studies by a team in England, the effects of essential oils from rosemary showed an increase in memory of 60–75 percent.[9]

In the mornings when my children left for school, I'd give them a sprig of rosemary or peppermint to put in their pocket. I'd tell them to smell it during the day for a lift or when they'd get ready to take a test. It was also a little something to remind them I loved them during their long hours at school. It still makes me smile to think about it.

Boredom is Not Such a Bad Thing

Did you know the author Jane Austen made up her amazing stories because she and her sisters were bored? When I read that, it occurred to me that children who were entertained all of the time by TV or video games were not encouraged to use their imagination to create their own music or stories. So I went wild with this idea, turning times that might have been boring into wonderful events of flourishing imagination. It may be one of the best things I ever did for my children.

For example, I planned trips to places where there was no TV, radio, or telephones. Although it challenged my husband, whose office would need to get hold of him, he made it work in those days before cell phones and email. Our family vacations allowed Amanda and Gibbons to feel confident and independent. They didn't always have to do something structured. As a result, they created wonderful board games, card games, stories, songs, and plays. How adventurous. Those were some of the happiest times in our lives.

Years later, my daughter served in the Peace Corps and lived in a mud hut in remote Mali, Africa with no electricity, running water, or internet connection. I believe these childhood experiences helped her handle this tough environment in a healthy way.

Learning to be alone and happy is a truly wonderful gift. It allows for room to think, be at peace, and have comfort in one's own company.

Adventures Away from Home

After our children got old enough, we enjoyed teaching them how to feel comfortable being away from home. Sometimes, we stayed at a hotel in our own city of Dallas. Gibbons and Amanda had fun riding in an elevator or an escalator, or ordering room service. When they were about four, we started taking trips overseas. Sometimes we would take my mother with us. Her presence made our excursions even more fun. We'd take turns staying in the hotel room at night when the children were asleep, so the other two adults could go out and see the city. We'd rent cars and drive across Europe.

One of the things I loved to do was buy a variety of age-appropriate books about the country we were going to visit. I did that for my benefit, too. It always made the trip more enjoyable, like a history lesson without effort. The children felt more compassion and excitement about meeting people in these countries after reading stories about children or animals who lived there.

On trips where we would have long days in the car, I would bring wonderful books on tape or CD, often about that country or maybe classics by authors such as Charles Dickens, James Joyce, Ernest Hemingway, or Emily Brontë. They made the long driving days more gratifying, and we loved to talk about the books later.

Listening is an art, and many people today don't really listen. I contend that listening for stretches of time trains a child to have a long attention span. In our family, we all benefited from reading wonderful books. I highly recommend this idea for anyone taking road trips!

Journal Writing

I also bought wonderful journals for writing and drawing. I encouraged Amanda and Gibbons to create a page for every day or place. Once, we accidentally left a journal behind in a hotel in Belgium. What a tragedy. That lost journal had been filled with beautiful drawings by my daughter from past trips, and the stories she had written were highly creative. After that, I always bought new journals for each trip. I wanted my children to have these journals when they grew up, so they could look back at how they'd experienced the world in their own words and pictures.

Writing in journals also gave them a quiet and reflective thing to do while waiting at the airport, train station, or hotel lobby. They learned to trust their inner voices and express themselves for their own enjoyment.

The link between the conscious and the unconscious is writing.

I read about a study that asked a group of teenagers to write down their life goals: what they'd be doing three, five, or ten years later.They followed these teens and found the ones who had written down goals were actually accomplishing them. The ones who didn't write down any goals or dreams or visions were unfocused and didn't tend to accomplish much. This is an easy and inexpensive exercise. Try doing this with your children, too! All you need is a journal or notebook for them to write in.

More Traveling Tips, Tricks, and Treats

I endeavored to think ahead when traveling with my children. I wanted to be ready for anything! So I packed simple, healthy food or snacks such as nut butter and bread that wouldn't spoil in case we got stuck where food wasn't easy to find. I'd include plain crackers for when they had a queasy stomach. Add ginger ale, and we had a home remedy.

We went to places such as India, Borneo, and Kathmandu where the spices or food were a little strong sometimes, and a bit unusual. Having a familiar sandwich from home made everything feel okay.

I would also pack a Ziploc baggie with my cleanse mixture, a teaspoon (for each of us for every day) of psyllium husks and raw green food powder. We'd carry it with us everywhere. Every day, I had Gibbons and Amanda take a teaspoon of this mixture in water or fruit juice, especially if we were somewhere exotic. The psyllium husks provided fiber and the green powder was high in antioxidants.

When traveling, people get all kinds of germs from various situations. The raw, green food powder, high in antioxidants, would flush out the bacteria and toxins; the psyllium husks would absorb the toxins and carry them out of the body. Getting the toxins out of the body is the key to a good cleanse.

Embracing this ritual cleanse kept us well and prevented illness or diarrhea. We started it when our children were about five, which is when I learned about it for the first time. They weren't always thrilled about it, but they drank it, and their health benefited from it. I did this cleanse with them at home, too.

I'd always pack an extra set of clothes including underwear, socks, and shoes for each of us in a carry-on. I included anything we couldn't do without for two days. Our luggage got lost at such odd times. If I hadn't packed like this on every trip, we would have been miserable. I still pack an extra carry-on of clothes to this day.

I also traveled with a deck of cards. We spent many an evening playing wonderful games of gin, hearts, Go Fish, or games the children would make up. What a relaxing way to spend time when the flight was delayed or everyone got tired of sightseeing. Our playing cards often became souvenirs from our trips.

Our type of souvenir was simple, such as playing cards or a T-shirt when we needed an extra sleeping shirt or a bathing suit cover-up. All these things made traveling fun!

Fostering Individuality

In today's world where mass media messages make fitting in so important, my children feel confident making their own decisions and being okay with being different. We always told our children not to follow the crowd but to march to their own drum. For example, my husband and I weren't fond of the idea of our son's being in a Boy Scout troop. I'm not criticizing the Boy Scouts. It's a wonderful organization. (My brother is an Eagle Scout.) It simply wasn't the right choice for our son at the time. We were concerned about fostering a "follow the pack" mentality, which can be similar to a gang mentality. Instead, we wanted our children to be leaders in making decisions on their own. We didn't want them to feel like they had to follow the crowd to be okay.

While it's fine to listen to the ideas of others, it's important to come up with original decisions and feel confident enough to move forward with them. In his career as a trial lawyer, my husband had to think on his feet and disseminate information in a fast and sometimes life-altering moment, making him agile at coming up with ideas, facts, or important information. This type of work was a part of our lives. Because of my husband's love of learning and thinking fast, he invented his own version of trivia that he played with the kids at meals and/or when traveling. He'd pick a subject related to our location, or art, or history, or whatever seemed right. This taught them to think fast while instilling the feeling that learning can be exciting, fun, and rewarding—without winning prizes. We never kept a running tally; each game proved to be a unique experience that gave us all a new start.

Whatever the weather may be, says he
Whatever the weather may be,
It's the songs ye sing,
an' the smiles ye wear
That's a makin' the sun shine everywhere.

—James Whitcomb Riley

CHAPTER 2

Dietary Aspects of Raising Healthy Children

As I began raising my children with a whole grain, organic, vegetarian diet, I was confronted by highly skeptical attitudes from family and friends. I voraciously read everything I could on food, nutrition, and health. I had all of our blood tested yearly for any signs of anemia or deficiencies. When I became a vegetarian, I stopped being anemic after a couple of years. Ironically, after a life of being forced to eat meat, I found that a healthy vegetarian diet *healed* me. I was amazed.

What's more, my children rarely got sick. When they were nine or ten, the pediatrician told me they were the healthiest children he'd ever seen. I felt elated. I'd come a long way since they were born.

After my son was born, I had not lost all of the weight I had gained during back-to-back pregnancies. Being about 50 pounds overweight and miserable, I took ballet classes and began eating healthier. A magazine called *Vegetarian Times* provided up-to-date news on health products and different points of view during this lonely transition to eating a plant-based diet. I bought health-related cookbooks and experimented with different cultural cuisines. Although I'm not advocating everyone be a vegetarian, I found that eating a mostly plant-based diet worked for me and my family at the time and continues to do so.

Years later, I took a plant-based nutrition class with T. Colin Campbell at Cornell University and learned about the China Study, considered to be the most comprehensive nutrition study to date. He said the study found when people have too much animal protein in their diets—whether from meat, fowl, fish, or dairy—tumors can form. This explains why a vegetarian diet can be healthier than a regular diet. This class revealed many studies proving people can overcome illness on a plant-based diet. Additional studies I've read since then have confirmed that.

For example, according to McGill University's website, studies show people on healthy vegetarian diets have "lower risks of coronary artery disease, colon cancer, hypertension, and diabetes and lung cancer."[11] In *Prevent and Reverse Heart Disease*, Dr. Caldwell B. Esselstyn, Jr., former president of the medical staff at the Cleveland Clinic, wrote about reversing heart disease with no drugs and only a plant-based diet.

> Based on the groundbreaking results of his 20-year nutritional study—the longest study of its kind ever conducted—this book explains, with irrefutable scientific evidence, how we can end the heart disease epidemic in this country forever by changing what we eat. Dr. Esselstyn convincingly argues that a plant-based, oil-free diet cannot only prevent and stop the progression of heart disease, but also reverse its effects.[12]

Walter Kempner, MD, founded the Rice Diet program. He believed that a diet of rice, fruit, and vegetables did miraculous things for people trying to regain their health. According to a lecture by John McDougall, MD, Dr. Kempner treated hundreds of people at Duke University. There, he prescribed a diet of rice, vegetables, and fruit that reversed hypertension, diabetic funduscopic changes, heart failure (cardiomegaly and EKG changes), kidney problems, and obesity.[13]

In the book *The China Study,* Dr. Campbell and his co-authors advocate a plant-based diet as a platform for optimum health. The following précis summarizes what he told our class at Cornell University:

> Plant-based eating is a superior way of eating. By eating this way, people can live longer, look and feel younger, have more energy, lose weight, lower their blood cholesterol, prevent and even reverse heart disease, lower the risk of prostate, breast, and other cancers, preserve their eyesight in later years, and prevent and treat diabetes. They can avoid surgery, vastly decrease the need for pharmaceutical drugs, keep bones strong, avoid impotence, avoid stroke, prevent kidney stones, prevent infants from getting type II diabetes, alleviate constipation, lower blood pressure, avoid Alzheimer's, beat arthritis, and more.[14]

About studies on populations where meat protein was introduced into the diet, Dr. Campbell said his early research gave him the understanding that animal protein, when tested experimentally, was substantially different from plant protein in its ability to promote tumor development.[15]

More than 100 million people today have diabetes or pre-diabetes. A recent study conducted by a team of American and Japanese researchers showed that people who have diabetes can vastly improve their health by eating an entirely plant-based diet.[16] This agrees with my experience. During my work with people who have diabetes, I have found they show remarkable improvement in their health from consuming a plant-based and almost completely raw diet.

Along with this research is a new meta-analysis in which these researchers compared six significant prior research studies. The researchers found a plant-based diet significantly improved blood sugar control in type 2 diabetes and specifically in a key indicator of blood sugar control called hemoglobin A1c. The participants' results improved as much as 1.2 points, which is greater than the effect when typical oral diabetes medicines are used.[17]

The study also focused on combining the results of all of the available studies. It indicated the benefit of excluding dairy (including cheese), eggs, and meat from the diet was as much as 0.7 points in some studies, averaging 0.4 points overall.[18] Considering long-term effects, note that the participants in most of these studies were not required to reduce their calorie or carbohydrate consumption.

However, I allowed my children to eat the food they wanted when they were at school or away from home. My son, now in his late twenties and over six feet tall, started eating meat later in life, while my daughter remains a vegetarian.

What I do know is everyone needs to find what works best for them and find balance in their life. I also know that the quality of the food is vital. From my studies, I believe an organic, plant-based diet can benefit your health and even heal your body.

Enlisting the Family in Making Meals

It was not always easy to get everyone in the family to try my new dishes. But, I discovered if I enlisted my children's help in the shopping, preparation, and presentation, they got excited about trying the new meals.

One night, I had my children and husband each decide on one dish they would make themselves, alone, as part of our family meal. I had them each find a recipe and let me know what they picked, so we didn't have two of the same dish. When all were completed, we'd enjoy them together as our meal. We each picked out our recipe, and then we went to the supermarket together to individually shop for the ingredients of our chosen recipe.

Our discussions were enlightening and fun. The children learned how to pick out food for a recipe as well as shop at the grocery store. When we got home, we had fun preparing our dishes separately but together in the kitchen. Then we all sat down and enjoyed our terrific meal. This was such a fun experience we did it again and again!

> *My son would inevitably pick out a super simple dish such as glazed carrots. Those carrots were some of the yummiest I've ever eaten! Everyone loved tasting each other's creations. It was one of the most delicious quality times we've ever had at a family meal.*

Today, my children love to cook and make delightfully delicious meals for themselves and their families. One day, my son's wife told my daughter that she loves going to the grocery store with Gibbons because he takes time to read and buy quality ingredients. They love cooking together. When I visit, they always have a delicious meal planned for us to prepare and enjoy together.

CHAPTER 3

Environmental Aspects of Raising Healthy Children

Having been married to an environmental lawyer for 23 years, I've learned a lot about air, water, farming, chemicals, concentrated animal environments, building materials, radiation, landfills, electromagnetic fields, and recycling. At times, I wish I didn't know what I do. It can be depressing.

That said, I have learned about toxins and problems with our buildings and environment. So we wouldn't feel helpless, the children and I wrote letters to groups or organizations. We wanted to become a part of the solution instead of believing there was nothing we could do. We also volunteered when we could. I started the Environmental Club at their middle school as the parent leader. Students and parents together planted wildflower seeds and set up recycling awareness programs. Years later, my daughter implemented recycling at her sorority house at the University of Texas.

The Plight of the Bee

Because I love reading environmental, gardening, and wildlife articles and books, I became aware of the plight of the bee 27 years ago. It makes me sad that it's only now becoming a widely recognized issue. The large bumblebees were becoming extinct over 28 years ago because the genetically engineered plants had flowers without nectar. Bees were starving to death.

Over time, I noticed more and more flowers in florist shops and gardens didn't have a fragrance. No fragrance, no nectar. What a shame. I love the fragrance, and I love the bees.

Our web of living depends on every little aspect of life. When one is taken out, it can start a downward spiral. Bees are natural to our environment, and our lives depend on our environment so much. Genetically engineered plants are escaping into the wild and interbreeding with wild plants. I am alarmed at the possible repercussions for the future of our earth and the future of our children's and grandchildren's food.

In 2012, an article in *Forbes* magazine stated it's not surprising bees are dying off in huge numbers because of the increase in genetically modified foods. "As of 2012, it is estimated that over 70 percent of the food on the U.S. market contains genetically modified organisms, ingredients that have been scientifically engineered in laboratories."[19] The article goes on to say, "These GMOs are not to be confused with produce items such as tangelos, pluots, and grapples, which come to be through a process of cross-breeding, and not laboratory-conducted genetic engineering."[20]

GMO Foods Tested

Why are GMO (genetically modified organism) foods harmful? Tests feeding three types of GMO corn to rats showed these results:

> Effects were mostly associated with the kidney and liver, the dietary detoxifying organs, although different between the 3 GMOs. Other effects were also noticed in the heart, adrenal glands, spleen and haematopoietic system. We conclude that these data highlight signs of hepatorenal toxicity, possibly due to the new pesticides specific to each GM corn.[21]

During the tests, the rats also developed large tumors.

Taking Action

The combination of GMO plants, health risks, and the decline of the bee alarmed me so much I raised money for an organic hummingbird-butterfly garden at my son's elementary school. This would help educate the community about the importance of our pollinators. Today, the science, art, and English departments still use that garden. In fact, they are adding an organic food garden—all organic and free of GMOs—and teaching the children to be "master gardeners." I consult with them and Chip Clint, the organic gardener who designed the hummingbird-butterfly garden for the elementary school more than 15 years ago.

Elementary schools where children can work in the garden show students have much higher math and science scores than schools without gardens. It makes the children happy to have an outdoor science lab where they learn.

Given the enormous number of genetically modified and hybrid plants that lack nectar—and the growing amount of electromagnetic fields and radiation put out by cell phone towers, computers, and electrical lines—bees, other pollinators, and many living creatures on earth face extinction. What can we do?

We can plant wildflowers and heirloom flowers in the garden and avoid killing the pollinators. They are not the enemy. The heirloom and wildflowers, which are rich in nectar, will support pollinators as well as attract them into the garden. Even growing a few in pots on a patio can be fun and rewarding for children. It helps them grow their own food and understand our connection with the earth.

Money, Energy, and Kindness

One thing business has taught me is that it's all about *money, power, and energy*. Money and power usually win out over everything. Where money and power are concerned, many people don't care about the quality of life or welfare of humanity. This makes me sad. It also makes me admire caring people who stand up to make the world a better place—money or no money.

We are all connected.
When one of us hurts, we all hurt.

Lighthouse for the Blind Volunteer

For 15 years, I taught a pottery-making class at the Lighthouse for the Blind as a volunteer working with people who had lost their vision. From the time my children were babies, they were regularly passed from one blind person to another. The blind people loved to hold my children and my children loved to be held by them.

Many of the people were very poor and physically challenged. Sometimes I'd clean their apartments. Obviously, it's more difficult for blind people to tell when something is clean or not. Sometimes, depending on the closeness of the relationship, I'd take them groceries, or clothes, or help in whatever small way I could.

My children often came with me. They'd water plants or just visit, which made them quite accepting of people with differences. My children learned to love some of these people dearly, and we still remember them fondly.

I always told them that having money didn't make people smart or good. It just meant they had money. I also said that *not* having money didn't mean they weren't good or not smart. It just meant they didn't have money right then. Money was simply energy without any stigma of being good or bad. It was a part of our lives.

CHAPTER 4

Behavioral Aspects of Raising Healthy Children

As the children grew up, I encouraged them to learn various arts, including music, to help their brains develop in ways that otherwise might not happen. Music stimulates the brain in the region where we learn language, science, and math. Gibbons and Amanda also took piano lessons and guitar around age 10. If they loved it and kept it up, great! It gave them the opportunity to allow that part of their brains to have additional stimulation. It also provided activities that didn't require others.

My husband—an excellent tennis player—and I encouraged them to play tennis when they were young. This exercise helped them develop quickness and hand-eye coordination while exposing them to sunshine and fresh air. Playing tennis didn't require them to be a part of a group.

Yet they participated in team sports, too. Gibbons loved to play baseball and today plays on adult teams. He also volunteers with the Miracle League, which makes it possible for children with disabilities to enjoy playing baseball.

Peer Pressure to Be Popular

As our children got older and peer pressure set in, many other parents grew extremely concerned about whether or not their children were popular. They encouraged their children to be cheerleaders or hang out with the captain of the football team instead of letting them naturally find their place to best fit in.

I never wanted my children to believe they should be doing anything except what they wanted to do. I had a different perspective than most parents.

I often heard parents say to their teenagers, "Aren't you going to the party this weekend?" or "Do you have a date?" This immediately puts in their minds they should be going to the party. If they aren't invited, then they feel left out, which is one of the worst forms of pain for anyone. If they don't have a date, it suggests something could be wrong with them.

So on weekends, we'd always have something fun to do, whether we went to an art museum, my family farm, a special science museum or movie, or a weekend getaway my husband and I planned. We'd invite our children. This way, if they hadn't been included in an activity with their peers, they didn't feel like they were missing anything. They'd often have more fun with us anyway, so it was a win-win situation.

Our main rule was they were to take good care of themselves at all times. Our second rule was no matter what time, place, or situation, they were always able to get in touch with us. We would be there for them immediately. We were always there for them, regardless of the situation.

Showing this support and *unconditional love* is critically needed for children to grow up strong and independent. Otherwise, they'll always be looking for the love they seek in groups, gangs, and teams. If they feel they are *unconditionally loved*—the kind of love they don't have to earn—they carry this with them in their hearts all through their lives. It gives them confidence and a comfort in their souls that they are worthy of love. They feel accepted just the way they are. What a priceless gift!

Creative Solutions to Behavior Problems

At times, we needed to find a solution to a problem or situation. Punishments should be about making children be better people, lifting them up instead of breaking them down. For example, when my son was going through a tough time in high school, he yelled at me and said mean, inappropriate things. I told him, "Okay, you're going to the bilingual university in Cuernavaca, Mexico for a week as your punishment."

At this university, people learn Spanish individually, not as a group. This punishment meant he'd be on his own in a foreign country, go to school, and take care of himself. If this experience played out well, it would teach him confidence, self reliance, independence, and better Spanish—a good solution. When he yelled at me again, I said, "Okay, that makes it two weeks. Every time you yell at me, it will be one more week."

Students at this university stay with a host family to become immersed in the language and culture. There were many nice families to choose as hosts. But because I wanted this to be punishment, not a luxury vacation, I chose one of the less affluent ones. In this family, my son would have to do his own laundry, cook his own food, get himself up for school, and go there on his own.

Luckily, our family had enough money to implement a punishment like this. If yours doesn't, look around your own area for similar solutions.

Gibbons went to Mexico feeling a bit apprehensive, but he got into a rhythm with his host family. He made friends with the teenage son who taught him how to make incredible Mexican food. He learned Spanish and practiced it with family members. He also gained a sense of responsibility without his parents pushing or threatening him.

This punishment was one of the best I ever came up with. He came home a new young man, kinder and more patient. Plus, he made awesome Mexican food for our family, and his Spanish grades greatly improved. Helping him raise his consciousness to a higher level benefited our whole family.

When children get frustrated and act out, if we can get them out of that place, then everything can shift.

As a parent, I want to take the focus off my children's problems, given that their world naturally revolves around them. I'm not saying their perceived problems aren't important, but they can appear all-consuming when they don't have to be. The passage of time or a shift of perspective helps them see other avenues that aren't self-centered. That's why another punishment I suggest is having your child volunteer to assist less fortunate children. Tutoring homeless children after school or volunteering at blind services or another nonprofit organization are excellent opportunities.

If the place they volunteer wasn't one where I'd leave my children on their own, we'd make it a family event. After all, when one member of the family hits a tough time, all of us can share in the solution.

When children can see other children's lives compared to their own, they realize their problems aren't so big after all. It shifts their perspective, creates a new understanding of life, and often brings families closer together.

Helping others makes us feel capable, more fortunate, and empowered. Most importantly, it shifts a child's energy out of the "poor me" phase into another perspective on life.

Trusting and Learning Responsibility

As our children got into high school, at times they'd ask for an extended curfew or special privileges. I had my own way of looking at this type of request.

First, I knew they wouldn't ask unless it was important to them. Second, they needed to learn responsibility before going off on their own after high school. I responded to their requests, "Tell me why you need an extended curfew (or whatever special privilege it may be)." I'd listen to their reasoning—*really* listen, which is the key every time. Then I'd say, "Okay, you know your main rule." The number one rule in our family was, "Take good care of yourself."

After that, I'd make them repeat the main rule to me verbatim: "I will take good care of myself." Then I'd say, "I trust your judgment. I know you will make the right decisions for yourself. Yes, I trust you, and you may have your curfew extended."

In this way, I put the responsibility on them. I also gave them room to grow and be responsible for themselves. They discovered they could make good decisions that kept them out of harmful situations. More times than not, Amanda and Gibbons came home *before* their normal curfew time. They wanted to *bend over backwards* to prove my faith in them was rightfully placed. This helped them handle their own decision-making when they were first living away from home. As my daughter once told me, even after she had lived in Africa in the Peace Corps, the most dangerous time and place for a child is in college.

Over the years, my children have lived in many countries. Being in various decision-making roles has helped them take care of themselves and not get into situations that could cause them harm. They know being safe is ultimately their own responsibility.

Putting Things into Perspective

There are times when we have accidents or situations that trouble us. My children and I have experienced many throughout our lives, such as when they were learning to drive and got into accidents. They would be terribly upset, knowing it would be costly and time-consuming to repair the cars.

I would urge them to put everything into perspective. I'd ask, "Okay, what is the worst thing that happened? Did anyone get hurt?" Thankfully, in these instances, no one was hurt. "Only a car was hurt, right? Well, okay, it's just a car, a thing. It can be fixed. As long as you are all right, then everything is okay."

Or if they had to ask someone a question and were afraid to do it, I'd say, "Okay, what's the worst that could happen? Your request could be turned down. So now apply that to a school situation. Ask that teacher or counselor if you can apply for the position you want. Whatever it is, ask. If you don't, you'll always wonder if you should have or could have. Shoot for the stars. If you don't reach the stars, you may end up on the moon!"

Getting turned down isn't that bad. What's bad and sad is being afraid to try. Looking at things with a new perspective can help immensely. If you put terrible or overwhelming situations into a positive perspective, you can help your children move forward without beating themselves up.

Peace of Mind is Priceless

At times, my children faced tough decisions. It could be two friends who weren't getting along, with my child caught in the middle. Often, there was no clear-cut decision as to which side to take. But, my approach was that there's always one choice that's the "right" choice, or at least closer to right than any other.

When we face decisions that weigh heavily on our minds, we can feel overwhelmed. I'd tell my children to look at their choices and ask,

"Which one would allow you to sleep peacefully at night? Which one would bring peace of mind to you? Then that's the decision to make."

Why is that a good approach? Because in the long run, that choice will bring them better health and a happier life.

No matter how hard it is to make a choice, choosing health is always the right decision to make.

My studies on health and the body-mind communication taught me that many diseases result from emotional trauma. We may not always have direct control over those situations. But when we do, our lives will be much happier and healthier if we make a choice that brings true peace of mind.

I have always loved how my children could fall asleep immediately and sleep deeply and peacefully all night long. True health comes from true peace of mind. That is priceless.

The more that you read,
the more things you will know.
The more that you learn,
the more places you'll go!

—Dr. Seuss

CHAPTER 5

Nutrition—Where to Start?

Everyone wants to raise the healthiest children possible. I certainly did. I started researching health, food, and nutrition before my children were born. My children were breastfed and raised on homemade baby food. As they grew up, most of the meals they ate I prepared at home. I made double or triple portions, saving or freezing some for later.

As the children got older, I let them help me buy, prepare, and serve food. As grown-ups, Amanda and Gibbons love creating their own healthy dishes and have turned out to be wonderful cooks. A good deal of what they make is whole and organic.

The quality of the food is vitally important for growing children, especially up until the age of 22. What they eat becomes their organs, cells, and bones. Their food should be as organic as possible—without hormones, antibiotics, MSG, dyes, sulfites, synthetic sweeteners, sugar, toxins built into genetically engineered foods, refined and processed ingredients (such as flour, sugar or salt), or other chemical additives.

I also recommend using whole, sprouted, or gluten-free grains. If you can't avoid dairy products, only use high-quality, humanely raised, organic dairy, free of antibiotics and hormones. Starting around the age of four, humans lose the ability to digest lactose. After that age, adding more nondairy milk to the diet is a good option. You can also substitute goat's milk, which is easier to digest than cow's milk.

In addition, I suggest eating fresh fruits separately from other foods as often as possible. Because fruits break down quickly, they will digest more easily and efficiently when eaten without other kinds of food.

Basic Guidelines for Healthy Eating

- Consume foods which are free of GMOs and grown without pesticides or chemical fertilizers.
- Consume only whole grains when eating anything made from grain (e.g., pasta, bread, crackers, chips) and avoid corn and wheat (especially genetically modified varieties). Gluten-free, sprouted, whole grains are preferred.
- If weight is a concern, eliminate corn and wheat completely.
- Consume no sugar or as little as possible. Take in no more than 15 grams a day. One teaspoon of sugar shuts down the immune system for five hours, according to Dr. Cynthia Champion-Olson, board-certified traditional naturopath and clinical nutritionist, and the *American Journal of Clinical Nutrition*.[22]
- Sugar is addictive. Avoiding it avoids the addiction.
- Do not use synthetic sugar substitutes in any way, shape, or form. (I discuss aspartame later in this chapter.)
- If a sweetener is absolutely necessary, try xylitol, stevia, dates, or (for older children) raw, organic honey. These are the most natural.
- Get enough protein each day from a variety of non-animal proteins. Lentils, beans, seeds, nuts, and leafy greens are terrific ways to consume the recommended amount of plant-based protein.
- Consume only quality, plant-based fats that support brain health and boost energy. Get enough of the essential fatty acids omega-3 and 6. Some high-quality, plant-based omega-3 fats include cold-pressed, organic hempseed or flaxseed oil, which must be kept refrigerated in the store and in your home. Another plant-based fat that supports overall health is pure, organic coconut oil.
- Include all of the B vitamins, especially B6 and B12, in a whole food base. That way, your body can easily absorb and use them. If buying a supplement, use one that comes from whole, organic foods instead of derived from chemicals.

- Get enough iodine, vitamin D, magnesium, zinc, iron, and calcium. Do not overlook these all-important nutrients.
- Chew food thoroughly. Eat while you're sitting down and relaxed.
- Consume foods that are organic, whole, and fresh. Make fresh, enzyme-rich, or what some call "living or raw" whole foods a major part of your diet.
- Avoid foods that come in cans, containers, packages, wrappers, or through the car window. Avoid processed or fast foods.
- Do not drink liquids (especially cold liquids) with meals. They water down the digestive enzymes. We want the digestive enzymes in our gut to digest food as efficiently and easily as possible. Cold liquids shut down the digestive system for an hour and a half. Shutting down one's digestive system during a meal doesn't make good sense.
- Drink half of your body weight in ounces of high-quality water each day. If you weigh 140 pounds, drink 70 ounces of water daily. Make sure the water is electrolyte-rich and free of sugar and chemicals such as chlorine and fluoride. Chlorine and fluoride are carcinogens which also harm the thyroid gland. Sugar puts stress on the pancreas. It will also shut down the immune system, and it can turn into fat.
- Add spices—not sugar—to jazz up any dish. Spices can enrich your food while making it nourishing and delicious!

Children Copy Their Parents and Caregivers

Children don't always listen to what we say, but they watch what we do. They see the difference between *what is said* and *what is done.*

Although no one is perfect, you want to set the best example you can to teach your children about eating in a healthy way. Show you care about the quality of food and its preparation. Most likely, they'll adopt your healthy habits over time.

Be sure to eat in a calm, relaxed manner, chewing your food so well it's practically in liquid form when swallowed. This contributes to preventing acid indigestion. Acid indigestion or a nervous stomach can result from food that's gulped instead of chewed thoroughly. The result? Weight gain.

In France, when they eat, it's important, It is an *experience*. In the U.S., we tend to treat our food as fuel. We eat standing up, walking, sitting in our cars, or watching TV. We don't treat our food as something we savor and "experience."

Look at food as a treat as well as an important part of our lives and our health. When we slow down and really enjoy our food, what happens? We eat less. We digest better. We enjoy our food more. We cut down on stress in a huge way.

Drinks and Food for Health

Great health hinges on great digestion, thorough absorption of nutrients, and quick, complete elimination of waste from the body.

Instead of drinking *during* meals, children can drink fresh juices and water *between* meals. The best time to drink is two to two and a half hours before or after a meal. Room temperature drinks are preferable to cold drinks, which can shock the system and shut down the digestive system for about an hour and a half.

Drink one ounce of water or nutrient/electrolyte fluids for every two pounds of body weight per day. The fluid should be high-quality and might include *structured* water, coconut water, freshly juiced vegetables and/or fruits, or white or green tea without added sugar.

Fresh vegetable and fruit juices have wonderful hydrating nutrients and fluids. Take those foods and liquids into account when looking at how many fluids you need to drink that day.

Why Should Drinking Water Be Structured?

Water and its structure influence our health and well-being. For example, after studying water in a laboratory for 10 years at the University of Washington, Dr. Pollack has reported: "If you need an entity to function properly—take a muscle for example—if the muscle is not functioning, it's the protein and the water that are not functioning."[23]

Dr. Pollack's team is currently exploring how water gets de-structured. It's unclear whether boiling, for example, can de-structure it, or whether boiling might add structure. The flip side of the question is how to reintroduce structure to water. Two simple approaches to increase structure are:

- Cool the water to about 39 degrees F.
- Stir the water to the left, with a spoon, in a circular jar to create a vortex.

As Dr. Pollack says, "It does look as though when you reduce the temperature, this area of structure increases. In fact, we're studying the possibility that the structured water is actually an intermediate between water and ice."[24]

We also want our water to contain electrolytes. Filtering water, microwaving water, and changing water from its natural state directly affects characteristics such as electrolytes. Therefore, I recommend drinking only high-quality, electrolyte-rich, structured water for great health.

If the study of water molecules interests you, watch the movie *Water, the Great Mystery* and see Masaru Emoto's information and photographs at http://www.masaru-emoto.net/english/water-crystal.html.

Dairy Products and Health

Gabriel Cousens, MD, states in his book *There Is A Cure For Diabetes* that children with diabetic genetic tendencies who drink cow's milk have an 11–13 times higher rate of juvenile diabetes than children who are breastfed for at least three months. He notes cow's milk is the number one cause of food allergies among infants and children according to the American Gastroenterological Association.[25]

Many children have problems with obesity. Drinking milk may not help this situation. A cow is born weighing 100–200 pounds and naturally grows to 2,000 pounds in two years from drinking milk. Is this a desirable outcome for humans?

Did you know the human body handles goat's milk better than cow's milk? If a goat dairy producing organic, *unpasteurized*, raw products is nearby, look into purchasing its milk, yogurt, and cheeses. I say *unpasteurized* because when food is pasteurized, heat kills most or all the probiotics in it. With raw, unpasteurized products, the healthy probiotic properties remain intact.

Children lose the ability to digest lactose around the age of four. This effectively means everyone becomes lactose intolerant after that age. As a health-conscious parent, should you buy infant formulas that use soy instead of milk? Soy should be avoided as a milk substitute or a food unless it's fermented, as in soy sauce. Soy is known to disrupt hormones and prevent the body from absorbing other nutrients. It can be particularly harmful to males.

Consider these alternatives to soy and dairy: unsweetened rice, coconut, oat, quinoa, hemp, and nut milks. You can sweeten them yourself to taste more like dairy milk. I use xylitol or stevia liquid drops. A brand called SweetLeaf has a toffee-flavored stevia, and I use it in my milk alternatives. It tastes delicious.

Comfort Food

When our children are hurt or not feeling well, whatever we give them becomes "their comfort food." Many of my clients talk about what their parents gave them when they were hurt, sad, sick, or celebrating. They crave this food when they're having a tough day, feeling sad, or going through an emotional meltdown. It is their comfort food.

Comfort foods remind them of love they felt when they were taken care of by their parents or others. People commonly list cookies, muffins, cupcakes, ice cream, candy, sodas, white refined breads, or cakes. Not surprisingly, many who mention this are overweight, diabetic, and sick because of comfort foods. Even though they try to avoid eating comfort foods, their cravings remain strong.

It's best to start off on the right foot. Give children healthy treats that won't make them sick or overweight when they get older. Select organic, high-quality, freshly squeezed juices, fresh veggies or fruits, vegetable soups, or healthy smoothies. Make sure birthday cakes, bread, or pastas are whole grain, gluten-free, and low in sugar.

What are we really giving them? Our love. That's what they really connect with, not the unhealthy food. In the long run, they will love us for making the change!

Probiotics and the Immune System

The major part of the immune system is comprised of *microflora beneficial bacteria*, commonly referred to as probiotics. According to the World Health Organization and the Food and Agriculture Organization of the United States, probiotics are "live microorganisms, which, when administered in adequate amounts, confer a health benefit to the host."[26] Another name for probiotics is "friendly bacteria."

Why are probiotics important? The National Institute of Health website says, "Friendly or positive bacteria are vital for proper development of the immune system, to protect against microorganisms that could cause disease, and to the digestion and absorption of food and nutrients."[27] The widespread use of antibiotics has compromised the beneficial bacteria and beneficial flora in our bodies.

If you take antibiotics, they wipe out *all* bacteria, both good and bad. Good bacteria keep bad bacteria in balance. If you don't have any good bacteria or flora in your body to support your immune system, then it's compromised. Therefore, adding probiotic food is vital to the health and strength of your immune system.

Our lives have become saturated with antibiotics. They even reside in our water supply. Farmers are the top purchasers of antibiotics for their animals. Only buy meat, chicken, eggs, or fish that are free of antibiotics or hormones.

Using soap or antibacterial gel such as hand sanitizer is like taking an antibiotic. The antibacterial element from the soap or sanitizer is absorbed directly into the skin in the same way medicine on a skin patch goes right into your blood stream. This can kill the beneficial bacteria in the body, affecting your immune system the same way as oral antibiotics.

Because of the widespread saturation of antibiotics in our lives, we need to replenish these beneficial bacteria on a regular basis. Make these probiotic foods a daily part of your family's diet: Rejuvelac; garlic; onions; raw; unprocessed apple cider vinegar; raw, unprocessed, organic, non-GMO, unpasteurized, organic soy sauce. Try fermented quinoa, raw coconut kefir, cottage cheese, miso, tempeh, and fermented coconut products. You can easily make them with your children, who are more likely to consume these foods if they take part in making them. Here is a recipe for an easy, inexpensive, probiotic drink for you and your family. It's vegetarian and gluten-free. It's also vegan if you use apple cider vinegar insted of whey to soak the seeds.

RECIPE FOR REJUVELAC

Rejuvelac is a probiotic that you can drink easily. It's made with fermentation of seeds or grains. You can use other seeds, but the quinoa seed is a good choice because it's a complete protein and gluten-free. I received this recipe from the Optimum Health Institute when I attended its program.

I have changed this recipe a bit, because it doesn't address the phytic acid problem with the seeds. Due to the phytic acid, I add whey to the mixture and let the seeds soak for a day with the whey. That should eliminate the phytic acid.

An adult would drink about eight (8) four-ounce glasses a day (32 ounces). A child would drink four (4) ounces daily.

Ingredients:

1 c. of quinoa
3 T. organic whey (vegans can use apple cider vinegar instead)
3 cups pure non-chlorinated water
1 gal. pure non chlorinated water
1 gal. glass container
A small piece of cheesecloth
A large rubber band
1 large spoon

Directions:

1. Rinse the quinoa with running water. Rinse it until the water runs clear. (I place it in a small mesh colander or sieve to do this.)
2. Put the rinsed grain in the gallon jar with the whey and the 3 cups of water. Place the cheesecloth over the top of the jar. Put a rubber band around the top of the jar to hold the cheesecloth in place.
3. Let it sit overnight. Drain the water, the whey, and save the quinoa seeds and the cheesecloth.

4. Place the seeds back into the jar. Fill up the jar with the gallon of water.
5. Cover the jar top with the cheesecloth.
6. Place a rubber band around the top of the jar to hold the cheesecloth in place.
7. Stir the mixture once a day with the spoon and replace the cheesecloth.
8. Rejuvelac will ferment for about two days. After two days, pour out the mixture using a sieve or colander. Save the liquid. It is the Rejuvelac, the liquid probiotic, you will drink.
9. You can throw out the quinoa or use the quinoa immediately to cook; it will now be sprouted.

Notes:

1. You can use rye berries instead of the quinoa seeds.
2. Rejuvelac will last about a week in the refrigerator. If you are drinking 32 ounces a day, then this will last about four days. It is a little bitter or sour tasting—and smelly. It took me a while to get used to drinking it. I had it for the first time at the Optimum Health Institute, a wonderful alternative healing and rejuvenation institute with a genesis in Ann Wigmore's book The Wheatgrass Book. You can find an Optimum Health Institute in California and one in Texas.

Allergies and Immunizations

Many people develop allergies growing up. If your child has a reaction within 10–15 minutes of eating, drinking, or taking a medication or vaccination, note it immediately. Keep a list of things that create bloating, red blotches, pain, headaches, fever, or anything else unusual in your child's behavior. Keep a diary of these things, where they are, the date and time of day, and the city or location.

If you notice your child has a food allergy and you aren't quite sure of the source, have a blood test done. Find out what allergies he or she might have. For a list of safe foods that don't have certain ingredients like nuts or gluten, go to http://snacksafely.com/safe-snack-guide/.

When my children were young, only a few immunizations were customary. At the time, I didn't know I could refuse them for my children. Today, many more immunizations exist. I've read alarming information about their side effects and how children's immune systems are unable to handle them. See the interview by Joseph Mercola, MD, with Lawrence B. Palevsky, MD, FAAP, about immunizations: "Expert Pediatrician Exposes Vaccine Myths," November 14, 2009, www.Mercola.com. Also see Dr. Palevky in Resources.[28]

I recommend *Saying No To Vaccines: A Resource For All Ages* by Dr. Sherri Tenpenny, D. O., published June 16, 2008. This book is a comprehensive guide which explains how and why vaccines are detrimental to your and your child's health. Dr. Tenpenny is an internationally recognized expert and the first physician to offer documented proof that vaccines compromise the immune system. She substantiates her work with citations taken from Centers for Disease Control (CDC) documents and peer-reviewed journals offering irrefutable facts that fly in the face of information commonly regarded as truth in traditional medicine today.

The more educated we are, the more informed our decisions will be. In addition to immunizations, pesticides in buildings, yards, or parks are something to be aware of. Pesticides get absorbed through the skin and can cause neurological damage. Be careful you aren't exposing yourself and your family to chemical pesticides, too.

Role of Protein in Health

Protein is essential for maintaining healthy sugar levels in the blood, especially when eating carbohydrates. Protein, which is made up of amino acids, is a crucial part of building and maintaining cells and tissues. The body uses amino acids to make hemoglobin and insulin, which are necessary for maintaining health. Dr. Andrew Weil, says:

> I recommend that you divide your daily calories as follows: 40 to 50 percent from carbohydrates (including vegetables, fruit, whole grains, starchy roots and tubers, and legumes), 30 percent from fat, and 20 to 30 percent from protein, which amounts to between 100 and 150 grams on a 2,000 calorie-a-day diet.[29]

The RDA recommends 0.36 grams of protein for every pound of body weight, or 0.8 grams of protein for every kilogram. A 150-pound person should take in 54 grams of protein every day. Beans, seeds, leafy greens, legumes, grains, eggs, and dairy are all sources of protein. In fact, leafy greens are among the best sources of protein. Spinach is 45 percent protein.

Be aware of how much meat and cheese you eat, and limit it. According to the *American Journal of Clinical Nutrition,* "Cheese and beef elevate insulin levels higher than the dreaded high-carbohydrate foods like pasta."[30] When eating pasta, make sure it is 100 percent whole grain and preferably gluten-free. (See Resources in the back of the book.)

Soy Protein

Soy protein is a complete protein that can be hard to digest. The Chinese do not eat unfermented soybeans because they contained quantities of natural toxins or "anti-nutrients." In addition, they are high in phytic acid. Ingesting soy can keep the body from absorbing nutrients such as calcium, magnesium, copper, iron, zinc, and protein. According to Dr. Gregory Damato, "Soy can cause serious gastric and pancreatic distress, which can include cancer and deficiencies in amino acid uptake."[31] Soy also contains goitrogens—substances known to depress thyroid function.[32]

What soy food should you avoid completely? Soy isolate. This food is mostly processed in aluminum tanks that leach high levels of aluminum into the food. Frequently, MSG, flavorings, preservatives, sweeteners, and synthetic chemicals are added to soy isolate to get rid of the beany taste and add a meatier flavor. What happens? Test animals in experiments developed enlarged organs, particularly the thyroid and the pancreas.[33]

Soy should also be avoided because most of it comes from genetically modified (GM) seed. According to *Natural News*, "More than 95 percent of GM soy, and 75 percent of other GM crops, are engineered to tolerate glyphosate herbicide, the most common formulation of which is Roundup."[34] Roundup kills weeds, and it can kill cells in our bodies.

If you are eating noncertified organic foods, I highly recommend reading more about glyphosate herbicide. Beyond GM soy being sold as a food, it's also added to tortillas, breads, fake meats, and many other foods while touting a health benefit. Actually, soy is a cheap filler, not a health benefit. Read ingredient lists carefully.

Health and nutrition expert Dr. Joseph Mercola says the advertising industry has misled the public about the safety and health benefits of soy as well as its widespread use in the Asian diet. He states, "A study of the history of soy use in Asia shows that the poor used it during times of extreme food shortage, and only then the soybeans were carefully prepared (e.g., by lengthy fermentation) to destroy the soy toxins."[35]

Mercola cites a study about soy that did not say using soy was an optimum way to feed an infant. Rather, it explored the possible use of soy milk to feed infants whose mothers did not have sufficient milk in countries where cow's milk was not available. He noted that although a weak soy milk or "tofu chiang" was sold hot in Peking by street vendors for old people to use instead tea, it was not usual to feed soy milk to infants.[36]

Still, a billion-dollar industry supports and advertises soy as an answer to many health issues. For example, soy is frequently touted as being helpful to menopause, heart disease, and weight problems in women. Consider this from Medpedia: "Foods that contain at least 6.25 grams of soy, less than 3 grams of fat, less than 1 gram of saturated fat, and less than 20 milligrams of cholesterol can legally display an FDA-approved statement about soy's role in helping to lower heart disease risk."[37]

To address these health claims, two FDA employees, Daniel Doerge, PhD, and Daniel Sheehan, PhD, wrote a controversial letter of protest to their own employer in 2000. They protested the positive health claims for soy that the FDA was approving at the time.[38] They wrote:

> There is abundant evidence that some of the isoflavones found in soy, including genistein and equol, a metabolize[r] of daidzen, demonstrate toxicity in estrogen sensitive tissues and in the thyroid.
>
> This is true for a number of species, including humans. Additionally, isoflavones are inhibitors of the thyroid peroxidase which makes T3 and T4. Inhibition can be expected to generate thyroid abnormalities, including goiter and autoimmune thyroiditis. There exists a significant body of animal data that demonstrates goitrogenic and even carcinogenic effects of soy products. Moreover, there are significant reports of goitrogenic effects from soy consumption in human infants.[39]

Do a little research on the effects soy can have on the thyroid, one of our master glands that affects almost all aspects of our health, and estrogen. Furthermore, as far as soy isoflavones are concerned:

> For men, eating soy isoflavones can significantly reduce testicular function and lower luteinizing hormone (LH) production, which is what signals the testicles to work. A high soy intake and potentially lower level of LH increases the probability of estrogen dominance in men, contributing to hair loss, swollen and cancerous prostates, and insulin resistance. Dorris Rapp, MD, a leading pediatric allergist, asserts that environmental and food

estrogens are responsible for the worldwide reduction in male fertility.[40]

Soy can also create allergic reactions. In 1986, Stuart Berger, MD, placed soy among the top "sinister seven" allergens.

Now that you are aware of the facts, be skeptical when reading food labels or product packages that refer to the health benefits of soy. If you do buy it, purchase *certified organic* soy, because it doesn't come from genetically modified seeds. Or, buy sprouted and/or fermented soy for a more digestible and less harmful soy protein. *Always avoid soy isolates.*

Phytic Acid

Everyone knows that nuts, seeds, grains, beans, and lentils are very healthy for you and are full of nutrients. But many people don't know there is phytic acid in nuts, seeds, grains, beans, and lentils. This represents a serious problem in the modern diet. This acid can prevent the body from absorbing important minerals such as calcium, magnesium, iron, and zinc. It can cause acid indigestion.

It inhibits enzymes in your body, which are vitally important to digesting food properly. Phytic acid also has powerful anti-nutritional effects in a diet. The high level of phytic acid in these foods can result in many health problems including tooth decay, nutrient deficiencies, lack of appetite, and digestive problems.

Historically, indigenous cultures and farmers always soaked, sprouted, and prepared their seeds, nuts, grains, beans, and lentils properly to remove the phytic acid before consuming them or feeding them to animals. In modern society, this is not done, and the results can be detrimental to the health of people and their animals.

Because phytic acid is found in so many enjoyable foods, it is vitally important to understand this and always prepare foods in a way that removes or neutralizes this acid as much as possible. My recipes frequently include directions for removing the phytic acid from certain foods to make them easier to digest and provide the maximum nutritional value.

Raw and Living Foods

Raw and living foods are foods that have not been heated over 105–118 degrees F. The enzymes in the food retain much higher nutrient levels in this form. *It is all about enzymes.* We need them for digestion and nutrient absorption. Live enzymes in foods help us digest efficiently and completely. Remember, the key to health is a clean and nutrient-rich body.

Raw and living foods are the best form of foods for optimum health and wellness. These foods will feed the body on a deep, cellular level without stressing it as much as cooked food does. Cooked foods are dead. They don't supply any live enzymes.

When foods are devoid of living enzymes, it means the body has to work much harder and supply more of its own enzyme store to digest the foods. Pulling enzymes from storage and using them to digest enzyme-empty food makes the body work harder compared to eating foods that supply their own enzymes ready for digestion.

In addition, raw and living foods have more nutrients available for the body during digestion. One of the most vital nutrients is sulfur, which is often overlooked. Sulfur is critical to our body's metabolism, specifically the catalytic function of large numbers of enzymes. Without the proper levels of sulfur, our bodies aren't able to build good healthy cells, and this leads to illness.

Although sulfur is present in most organically grown fresh food, it is mostly found in fruits, vegetables, and some grains. Due to its unstable nature, the sulfur is quickly lost from food when it is processed, cooked, or stored. That's another reason having a diet that's high in freshly picked, raw, unprocessed, whole, organic food is vitally important.

Raw, living, unprocessed foods are also highly alkalizing. The body's pH (acidic balance) should ideally be 7.2 to 7.3. However, most people with chronic or acute diseases usually have overly acidic bodies with pH reading well below 7.3. Eating foods that are highly alkalizing can help the body maintain a healthier pH.

What kinds of foods are found in a raw and living food diet? Uncooked (not heated over 105 degrees F) and unprocessed fruits, vegetables, nuts, seeds, and grains make up this diet. Fruit is a pure form of food that digests quickly compared to other foods.

Many people have started eating raw foods to heal their bodies and be healthier. But be careful. If eating raw is taken to extremes, it can create an imbalance in the body and cause stress on the thyroid, spleen, and pancreas. Watch for foods such as spinach and Swiss chard that have oxalic acid. Oxalic acid can be hard on the body if taken in large amounts. More than that, it can prevent the body from absorbing other nutrients, like calcium.

What else can bring more balance to your body? Three things:

1) Eating a diet which varies the amount of raw food intake
2) Eating with the seasons
3) Eating lighter raw foods in the warmer months

If you add warm foods to your diet in the cool months, this can be supportive to certain parts of the body. For instance, the thyroid is better supported when cruciferous vegetables such as broccoli and cauliflower are lightly steamed or sautéed instead of eaten raw. This is because these foods—as well as yams, canola, and soy—contain natural chemicals called goitrogens that can interfere with thyroid hormone synthesis. Lightly steaming or cooking these vegetables deactivates these chemicals. Adding foods like cooked whole grain rice can work as a tonic for the spleen and pancreas.

A diet with a ratio of about 80 percent raw to 20 percent cooked food will work for most people throughout most of the year.

When I was breastfeeding, I noticed I made more milk when I was eating a lot of fresh greens. All the animals that make large amounts of milk eat fresh greens daily. So, it made sense to me to be a "grazer."

Enjoy your raw foods, but listen to your own body and be mindful of how they affect your children's bodies. Your goal is to create balance in their health, their diet, and their lives, too.

Best Salt To Use

"Without salt, life itself would not be possible."[41]

The word *electrolyte* is a medical term for salt. Humans need electrolytes to be healthy, yet most people are electrolyte or mineral deficient. Baby boomers grew up using white, refined, processed salt, which is 98 percent sodium chloride with added bicarbonates, chemicals, sugar, and preservatives. Iodine—the main nutrient that supports our thyroid gland—is added to many refined salts. However, it has insufficient iodine to prevent thyroid illnesses or provide for the body's iodine needs.[42] That said, iodine dissipates after being exposed to oxygen, making this type of salt an unreliable source of iodine.

Most conventional medical doctors don't differentiate between white refined salt and unrefined, mineral-rich sea salt. Yet white refined table salt is lacking in numerous minerals that are found in whole, natural sea salt.

Many food sources today are deficient in vital, dense minerals and nutrients. Soils are depleted, and refining and processing take out many or all of the nutrients in the foods. When we sweat, our bodies can lose many of the minerals in natural, unrefined, whole sea salt. These minerals must be replenished. Sea salt can also help balance the body by alkalizing it and helping restore a healthy pH.

Salt cravings signal a depletion in nutrients, minerals, and electrolytes. Salt cravings also signal that your thyroid and adrenal glands need minerals. If you have been craving salt or you're under a good deal of stress, have your thyroid checked. You want to make sure you're getting enough iodine in your diet.

Dr. Brownstein says low-salt diets promote toxicity and have:

> . . . adverse effects on numerous metabolic markers including promoting elevated insulin levels and insulin resistance. Low-salt diets have been associated with elevating normal cholesterol and LDL cholesterol levels, which in turn, have been associated with cardiovascular disease. Finally, low-salt diets will lead to mineral deficiencies and the development of chronic disease.[43]

We don't have many food sources for iodine, and it can be extremely important to our health. A 1994 study in the *British Medical Journal* reported that of 100 men and women between 55 and 75 who had mild to moderate hypertension, when common table (refined) salt was replaced with mineral salt high in magnesium and potassium, a reduction in blood pressure occurred. That reduction was equivalent to taking blood pressure-reducing drugs.[44]

According to Dr. Brownstein, salt in itself isn't bad. In fact, unrefined sea salt is important for life. But refined salt can be harmful. Choosing mineral-rich, unrefined sea salt promotes:

- the proper balance for the endocrine, adrenal and thyroid glands to function properly as well as supporting healthy blood pressure,
- detoxification of the body, and
- optimal functioning of the immune system, hormonal system, and cardiovascular health.

Various Sugars

We find sugar everywhere, presented in the most beautiful, innocent ways supported by societal norms. When my children were young, I tried my best to avoid giving them sugar or sweets, but this practice was sabotaged almost daily. For example, their grandparents would give it to them, and my friends would share goodies with them. I was actually called evil, cruel, or mean for not wanting my children to participate in Halloween and other sugar extravaganzas. But these simply weren't good messages for my children. It was extremely hard to stand up for my beliefs without wondering if I was depriving my children of a "good" childhood—good being a relative term.

I did well at the time, but I could have been stronger. In the end, I strongly believe in drawing lines concerning our own children and sticking to what we believe is right.

As humans, we're hardwired to eat sweet food. Back when humans were hunter-gatherers, sweet foods made us believe they weren't poisonous. Because of this, we are naturally inclined to sweet foods. Yet according to studies, sugar is four times more addictive than drugs like heroin.[45] Keeping sugar out of the diet and out of the house is a smart move. Doing so can actually *prevent* many health problems. Eat food that's sweet enough by itself, especially fruits and vegetables that are naturally sweet.

Did you know that over a period of two weeks, humans develop new taste buds for whatever they consume? So, if you give your children sugary foods, they'll develop taste buds for it and crave them.

At a birthday party for a one-year-old boy, I admired the beautiful cake, so perfectly designed and sparkly. After blowing out the candle, the little boy was given a piece of cake. As he was eating it, the father said to him, "Well, you aren't going to want to eat your vegetables after this." That's where it starts! These kind, educated, nurturing parents mean well. But what are they setting their children up for?

I suggest avoiding sugar as much as possible. If you *must* use sugar, select healthier kinds. You'll find a few dessert recipes that can be a healthier choice when you crave something sweet. I like to use dates in their natural form when I need a recipe to be sweeter. Dates are high in vitamin B. If I have to serve dessert, dates or raisins can fill the need for sweetness.

Avoid synthetic sugars and sugar substitutes altogether. Chemically derived sweeteners can have many harmful effects on health. Over time, they are toxic and indirectly lead to weight gain. They are also addictive and amplify the craving for sugar—the direct opposite result of why many people consume them.

For example, aspartame (found in 6000+ products) gets converted to formaldehyde in the body. According to the government department of Occupational Safety and Health (OSHA), formaldehyde is a carcinogen that can seriously harm your "liver, kidney, spleen, pancreas, brain, and central nervous systems."[46] In addition, formaldehyde can cause allergic sensitization and cancer. "The occupational health hazards of formaldehyde are primarily due to its toxic effects after inhalation, after direct contact with the skin or eyes by formaldehyde in liquid or vapor form, and after ingestion."[47]

Given a choice between high-fructose corn syrup and artificial sweeteners, high-fructose corn syrup is a better choice, although the choice is essentially between consuming a poison or an even worse poison.[48]

Artificial Sweeteners

Aspartame makes up the artificial sweeteners NutraSweet, Equal, Spoonful, and Equal-Measure. It is composed of three chemicals: aspartic acid, phenylalanine, and methanol.

Aspartame can cause many problems, including neurological ones. For example, "When the temperature of aspartame exceeds 86 degrees F, the wood alcohol in aspartame converts to formaldehyde and then to formic acid, which in turn causes metabolic acidosis. The methanol toxicity mimics multiple sclerosis; thus, people may be misdiagnosed with having multiple sclerosis. Multiple sclerosis does not lead to death whereas methanol toxicity does."[49]

According to a report from the National Institutes of Health,

"Methanol is extremely poisonous. As little as two tablespoons can be deadly to a child. About 2 to 8 ounces can be deadly for an adult. Blindness is common and often permanent despite medical care. How well the person recovers depends on how much poison is swallowed and how soon treatment is received."[50]

Aspartame is a Serious Issue

> Both the U.S. Air Force's magazine *Flying Safety* and the U.S. Navy's magazine *Navy Physiology* published articles warning about the many dangers of aspartame. They included the cumulative deleterious effects of methanol and the greater likelihood of birth defects. The articles note the ingestion of aspartame may make pilots more susceptible to seizures and vertigo (US Air Force 1992). Countless other toxicity effects have been reported to the FDA (DHHS 1995), other independent organizations (Mission Possible 1996, Stoddard 1995), and independent scientists (e.g., 80 cases of seizures were reported to Dr. Richard Wurtman, Food in 1986).
>
> —from "Reported Aspartame Toxicity Reactions."[51]

Examples of aspertame toxicity reactions can be found on the ASpertame (NutraSweet Toxicity Info Center web page at http://www.tiac.net/users/mgold/aspartame.

Frequently, aspartame toxicity is misdiagnosed as a specific disease. This hasn't been reported in the scientific literature, yet it has been reported countless times to independent organizations and scientists. In other cases, it has been reported that chronic aspartame ingestion has triggered or worsened certain chronic illnesses. Nearly 100 percent of the time, the patient and physician assume these worsening conditions are a normal progression of the illness. Sometimes that may be true, but many times it is chronic aspartame poisoning.[52]

According to researchers and physicians studying the adverse effects of aspartame, the following list contains a selection of chronic illnesses that may be caused or worsened by the chronic, long-term ingestion of aspartame.

Note: In some cases such as MS, the severe symptoms mimic the illness or exacerbate the illness but do not cause the disease. Also, please note that this is an incomplete list. Clearly, ingestion of a slow poison is not beneficial to anyone who has a chronic illness.

Brain tumors
Multiple sclerosis
Epilepsy
Chronic fatigue syndrome
Parkinson's disease
Alzheimer's
Mental retardation
Lymphoma
Birth defects
Fibromyalgia
Diabetes
Arthritis (including Rheumatoid)
Chemical Sensitivities
Attention Deficit Disorder [53]

Labeling: A Real Concern

Avoiding artificial sweeteners in any amount would be wise. Stick with real, whole, unrefined, or unprocessed sugars. Read ingredient labels carefully, and check for any sugar or sugar substitute.

Sadly, the labels are not always reliable. The Food and Drug Administration (FDA) allows artificial sweeteners to be added to such foods as dairy products without stating the name of the artificial sweetener on the label if it is added under a certain percentage. This lets manufacturers claim the product has fewer calories and less sugar than similar products. This should not be allowed! *All ingredients should be listed on the ingredients label. Period.*

It's a trick to make consumers think that fewer calories, less sugar, or "low fat" is healthier. Actually, adding harmful ingredients is worse than full fat or natural calories in food. We need to demand full disclosure of what's in our food. If we don't demand it, then it won't happen. We consumers should be able to know what's in our food supply. Let our voices be heard. That is the only way lawmakers know we even care.

Safe Sweeteners

Xylitol

One sugar I've used over the years is xylitol, especially if a recipe calls for granulated sugar. Xylitol is a sugar alcohol naturally found in fruits and vegetables. It's usually made from birch tree bark and other hardwood trees. Some sources say xylitol was discovered by German scientist Emil Fisher in 1891. When Finland had severe sugar shortages during World War II, people started making it commercially. After the war, Finnish dentists noticed that schoolchildren had unusually strong, cavity-free teeth. This discovery led the Finnish government to be the first to officially endorse the use of xylitol as a sweetener.

By the 1960s, Germany, Switzerland, Japan, and the Soviet Union were using xylitol as their preferred sweetener for diabetics. It was also used as an energy source for infusion therapy with patients who have impaired glucose intolerance and insulin resistance.

Xylitol is considered a five-carbon sugar, which means it has antimicrobial effects, preventing the growth of bacteria. It is also alkaline-enhancing and can replace sugar in recipes in equal substitution. Xylitol tastes and looks just like sugar with no bitter aftertaste.

Drug interactions have not been found. The only side effect is that when consumed in large doses over 30 or 40 grams at one time, it can cause gas and diarrhea. Some types of xylitol have a little bigger granule size than refined sugar. When purchasing xylitol, the smaller, finer grain variety will bake easier.

Xylitol and stevia are both sweeteners that can be used in diabetic diets. In addition to helping prevent cavities, xylitol can help repair dental enamel, regulate blood sugar for those with type 2 diabetes, strengthen bones, decrease age-related bone loss, inhibit serious systematic yeast problems, inhibit the growth of bacteria that cause middle ear infections in young children, inhibit the growth of streptococcus pneumonia, and alleviate dry mouth. It even inhibits inner ear and other infections. Mothers love that!

In addition, xylitol has 40 percent fewer calories and 75 percent fewer carbohydrates than sugar. It's slowly absorbed and metabolized, which results in negligible changes in insulin. Its consumption can reduce sugar cravings and insulin levels, and help alkalize your body. It was approved by the FDA in 1963.[54]

Stevia

Stevia is a sweetener derived from *Stevia rebaudiana Bertoni*, a South American plant in the aster family. Japanese food manufacturers developed this sweetener in the 1970s as a zero-calorie sugar. The Japanese have done extensive research on stevia and found it to be extremely safe. The less-refined varieties of stevia are the best in terms of health benefits. Less-refined foods of any type are healthier than refined ones because they are in a more natural, whole-food form.

Stevia comes in powder and liquid form. I have been using this sweetener for years. I like the liquid form best, because I think it has a better flavor, while the powdered form can be a bit bitter.

Honey

I love honey. Besides boosting energy, this natural sweetener is antifungal and antibacterial, so it can be used as a natural antiseptic and remedy for many ailments. It can even facilitate muscle recuperation and glycogen restoration after a workout.

Raw, unfiltered honey is a natural source of B1, B2, B3, B5, B6, and vitamin C. It has a variety of nutrients and minerals including magnesium, potassium, calcium, sulfur, and phosphate as well as some enzymes.

Honey can be substituted for sugar in recipes. However, make absolutely sure it's unprocessed and raw. Most honey in the U.S. today has been refined and processed, so it doesn't have the beneficial pollens that help reduce allergies. *Weekly World News* listed arthritis, hair loss, bladder infections, upset stomach, indigestion, influenza, longevity, heart disease, colds, and cholesterol as some of the afflictions that could be cured by honey and cinnamon.[55] Always buy raw, unrefined honey, because it will have all of the live enzymes and nutritional properties still intact.

Honey and Babies

Be sure to avoid giving an infant 18 months or younger honey or products made with honey. This sweetener sometimes contains trace amounts of botulinum spores. These are easily denatured by the mature digestive tract of an adult, but they can be harmful or even fatal to an infant whose digestive tract is still developing.[56]

Soul Food

Although what we consume feeds the body and soul, there is more to it than that. At the nutrition school I attended, Joshua Rosenthal taught us that we fill our body with things in life other than food. If we are eating well, but miserable in our relationships, job, or living conditions, that's not living a healthy life.

What people desire more than anything is food for the soul. Do your eyes light up when your child walks into the room? That's food for the spirit. Unconditional love is what everyone in the world seeks. When children don't get it, they spend the rest of their lives searching for love and acceptance. But when they get that unconditional love from a parent, they won't feel a need to find it elsewhere, such as in a group or a gang.

Remember, the main ingredient in any recipe is love!

When I was One,
I had just begun.

When I was Two,
I was nearly new.

When I was Three,
I was hardly Me.

When I was Four,
I was not much more.

When I was Five,
I was just alive.

But now I am Six, I'm as clever as clever.
So I think I'll be six now for ever and ever.

—A. A. Milne

CHAPTER 6

Babies and Breastfeeding, Children and Food

When we are born, we immediately bond with our mothers and with food. Nourishment helps form a strong family bond. My grandmother made the best food because she added the secret ingredient of love to her recipes. Food never tastes as good as when it is prepared with love. Many events and celebrations embrace the food we share. My clients tell me how they have struggled all of their lives to avoid eating foods like cookies, muffins, cake, and ice cream.

A mom wants to be a good mom, and she wants her babies to love her. So does a dad. When a child is ill or falls down and hurts his knee, many moms console their children by picking them up and holding them, showing love and comfort. Some may offer cookies, ice cream, or sweets to help the child stop crying or stop focusing on the pain. Many of my diabetic clients have said their mother gave them this type of food when they were hurt, sad, ill, or feeling upset. They say they have uncontrollable urges for these foods when they have a rough day or feel sad or lonely. These are their comfort foods.

What can you do differently? *In those times, offer your children foods that are healthy*. When they have a sore throat, give them a cool cucumber soup. When they are hurt, give them vegetable soup or a hummus sandwich. As they grow up, they will crave these foods when they want to feel comforted, foods that won't ruin their health.

When my children were babies, I breastfed them and started to make my own baby food. I would get high-quality organic vegetables or fruits and mix them with purified water in a blender or Cuisinart. How easy! I didn't want any sugar or additives.

There was no organic baby food in the stores when our children were infants. I had to make it myself if I wanted them to eat organic, unprocessed, living, or whole grain baby foods. I would also take the healthy meal I was making for me or my husband, then place it in a blender or food processor and puree it. When I made my own baby food, I knew exactly what was in it. I loved that!

A simple thing to do with baby food is putting it in small glass containers you refrigerate or freeze. You can have a simple snack or meal when you're on the go, or have it on hand for your children's caregivers if you work outside the home.

When children's bodies are growing, what food they eat is more critical than later in life because it helps form their organs. Any residue from pesticides and fertilizers concentrates more in a child's organ than in an adult whose organs are mature.

When I heard this, I took it seriously. I tried very hard to provide as much organically grown food for my children as I could. I had to order a lot of my food straight from the organic farms, because there were so few Dallas stores that sold organic foods back then. We started our own vegetable garden with heirloom seeds.

In addition, I didn't give my children any sugar at all for a few years, until I was really shamed into it by people who wanted to give them sweets for holidays. I didn't participate in Halloween until finally I gave into pressure from many people who thought I was depriving my children of a treasured childhood event.

Once my children entered school, it was harder to monitor their sugar intake. So I began to experiment with making healthy, whole grain xylitol treats. They were a little heavier than the white, refined types of sweets, but they had a depth, texture, and quality to them that made them rich. With time and frequency, they grew on us. Because we knew they were much healthier, it made it a better choice mentally as well. I would do this again in a heartbeat if the situation arose.

It was difficult for me to watch my children eat things I knew were bad for them, but I knew it was important for them to have friends and not be seen as the weird children with the weird mom. So, I did my best when I could. I still remember the phone call from my daughter when she had gone to a friend's home to play after school. She was panicked. "Mom, what do I do? She is taking us to McDonald's!"

I was so shocked. It had not occurred to me that this is what happened on play dates. We worked out that she would get an order of French fries and a glass of water. Now we know they were putting meat juice and all kinds of chemicals for flavoring in the fries. But at the time, it seemed like the least harmful thing to order. I'm still distressed that people commonly visit these fast food places. I'm also amazed when I go to a grocery store and observe the foods people buy. However, I can still be happy with my own choices.

I switched to fresh, organic, whole grain, mostly gluten-free, vegetarian food 27 years ago. It has been a learning experience and one that no doubt has made my family and me healthier. You do have to pick your poison, though. Not *everything* I choose is healthy. I do love to eat out, and we ate out a lot. So, we would simply order what was the best choice for us. It was a fun part of our social life. When we were at home, we could better control our food choices, but going out was a treat for us emotionally. Sometimes you just have to do the best you can and simply go with what the choices are in the moment.

The Benefits of Breastfeeding

One of my most cherished memories is the feeling I had when sitting in my babies' room, holding and nursing them, often in the still of the night. I loved looking at those tiny fingers wrapped around mine.

The first breast milk is made up of colostrum, which is rich in nutrients and antibodies that protect the baby. In contrast, formula feeding raises health risks in babies that might include:

- ear infections
- diarrhea
- necrotizing enterocolitis, a disease that affects the digestive system in premature infants
- lower respiratory infections
- asthma
- obesity
- type 2 diabetes

Moms benefit from breastfeeding, too. Life can be easier without having to deal with cleaning bottles and spending money on formula. Breastfeeding is both bonding and relaxing for mother and child.

Breastfeeding is linked to a lower risk of these health problems in women:

- type 2 diabetes
- breast cancer
- ovarian cancer
- postpartum depression

Many studies have reported greater weight loss for breastfeeding mothers than for those who don't breastfeed. Breastfeeding mothers miss fewer days from work because their infants are sick less often.[57]

The Surgeon General's Call to Action to Support Breastfeeding made this statement:

> Because breastfeeding confers many important health and other benefits, including psychosocial, economic, and environmental benefits, it is not surprising that breastfeeding has been recommended by several prominent organizations of health professionals, among them the American Academy of Pediatrics (AAP), American Academy of Family Physicians, American College of Obstetricians and Gynecologists, American College of Nurse-Midwives, American Dietetic Association, and American Public Health Association, all of which recommend that most infants in the United States be breastfed for at least 12 months. These organizations also recommend that for about the first six months, infants be exclusively breastfed, meaning they should not be given any foods or liquids other than breast milk, not even water.[58]

Experts are still looking at the effects of breastfeeding on osteoporosis and weight loss after birth.

What You Ingest Can Mean the Difference Between Life and Death

When you are pregnant or nursing, what you ingest directly affects your infant. I read an article about a woman whose physician had prescribed a painkiller after her child was born. The article said, "Codeine prescribed for postnatal pain can produce deadly concentrations of morphine in breast milk."[59]

A lawsuit over the death of Toronto newborn Tariq Jamieson, who died as a result of opiate toxicity in his mother's breast milk, has renewed the debate over prescribing such drugs as Tylenol 3 to breastfeeding mothers. Tariq's mother Rani was prescribed Tylenol 3 for lingering episiotomy pain. Although Tariq was initially healthy, he developed increasing lethargy after the seven-day mark, and after 11 days he was brought to a pediatrician due to concerns about his skin color and poor feeding. Two days later, Tariq died. As stated in the National Review of Medicine on June 15, 2007:

> Tariq was found to have high blood levels of acetaminophen, and a blood concentration of morphine six times higher than would normally be considered safe in a neonate. Tylenol 3 contains both acetaminophen and codeine, which is metabolized to morphine in the body. However, not everyone metabolizes codeine at the same rate. Rani Jamieson was an ultra-rapid metabolizer of codeine to morphine, which means that the opiate built up in her breast milk very fast.[60]

When I was breastfeeding and ate leafy greens, I had an abundance of milk. When you think about it, a cow eats greens all the time and they make a lot of milk. The greens are alkalizing and rich in nutrients—a great choice to have as a main part of the diet.

Breastfeeding is important for mother and child. But be careful about what you ingest, so you can protect your little one's fragile life.

CHAPTER 7

Ummm . . . The Sweet Taste of Breakfast

Breakfast is the most important meal of the day. But how often are we in a hurry and don't feel like preparing this meal or cleaning up afterward? Instead, many of us reach for cereal, protein or fiber breakfast bars, or other easy-to-prepare, easy-to-eat foods.

I grew up eating cereal and milk for breakfast, so I understand how simple and yummy it can be. Yet, I've since discovered these aren't the best choices. Why? Because many cereals on the market today can have high amounts of sugar, which is a main contributor to obesity, diabetes, and heart disease. In particular, I'm addressing *added* sugars, not those found naturally in fruits or whole unprocessed foods. When whole dried fruits are added to foods, they do raise the number of sugar grams, so be aware of that.

Our bodies simply don't handle sugar well. Sugar affects us like an addictive drug. It can even make us sick! According to Yale Health Newsletter, a child should be limited to 3–4 teaspoons of added sugar a day and an adult to 5 teaspoons a day. However, many people are taking in as many as 22–34 teaspoons of sugar a day.[61] (Note: Four grams of sugar equals one teaspoon.)

Here's a key problem with *any* amount of added sugar: According to the *American Journal of Clinical Nutrition*, one teaspoon of added sugar shuts down a person's immune system for up to five hours. So, if we feed our children a sugary breakfast and then send them off to school, what happens? Their immune systems can stop functioning efficiently shortly after they arrive in class. Is it any wonder they often come home sick?[62]

Which Cereals to Choose

I suggest purchasing only the highest quality cereal with the fewest number of additives. Sometimes my choice centers on budget or time constraints, but I certainly make the best choice I can in the moment.

Let's examine the array of available breakfast cereals and determine the healthiest choices based on their ingredients. The ingredients noted here include more than sugar content. Although sugar is the main ingredient to be mindful of, watch for other ingredients as well.

When you're grocery shopping, follow these steps:

1. Before leaving for the grocery store, take your reading or magnifying glasses and be prepared to read the lists of tiny ingredients on the packages.
2. When reading ingredient lists, look at how big a serving the packaging shows related to the amounts being analyzed. For example, some cereals show "½ cup" as the serving amount and others say "1 cup." If you are eating 1 cup and the amount measured is only ½ cup, you need to calculate double the amount of sugar stated in the serving. To compare products, you may have to do a little math, but it's worth the effort.
3. As you read the ingredients, notice if the grains are listed as whole grain or sprouted whole grain. Sprouted grains or seeds are easier to digest than whole grains.
4. Also read the front of packages, which can be quite deceiving. The descriptions can say the cereal contains whole grains, but it may hardly contain any whole grains at all. If whole grains are in the product, then the manufacturer can legitimately say so in large print on the front of the package. You have to check and make certain the ingredient list reflects what's being claimed on the packaging.
5. Take notice of the first 4–6 ingredients. They are listed by most to least of how much the product contains. If sugar is listed

among these first ingredients, you know the cereal is high in added sugar. Also notice what type of sugar has been added. Is it a high-fructose corn syrup, corn syrup, cane sugar, agave nectar, date sugar, rice syrup, molasses, fruit juice concentrate, xylitol, honey, or stevia? In my opinion the xylitol, stevia, and honey are less harmful as a sweetener than the others, so choose those options.

6. Notice if the product has *hydrogenated* oils. Any fat that's been hydrogenated or molecularly changed is called a trans-fat, which makes it a bad" fat in even the smallest amount. Never purchase a cereal with this type of fat listed in its ingredients.
7. Look to see if the list includes any natural flavorings, added food color, or preservatives such as BHT or BHA. The University of California's *Berkeley's Wellness Report* says to avoid these completely. Preservatives, color additives, monosodium glutamate or MSG (frequently listed as natural flavorings, spices, and hydrolyzed proteins) are also to be avoided. These types of additives have been linked to childhood behavioral problems and cause other types of health problems. [63]
8. Select the brand that has the least amount of sugar and the most whole grains or sprouted grains, preferably free from GMOs (genetically modified organisms).

Practice checking the specifics in the ingredients so you can make more educated and healthier choices for your family.

Sugar Content

I've compiled a short list of cereals, food bars, and nondairy milks with the grams of sugar listed for each one. This allows you to see how many of the apparently healthy cereals have high sugar content. Special note: Don't assume that because a product is found on the shelf in a "natural" grocery store that it's necessarily healthy.

Cereals with Lowest Amounts of Sugar

The following brands of cereal have the *least* amounts of sugar:

Ezekial 4:9 – Original	½ cup has 0 grams
Ezekial 4:9 – Almond	1 cup has 2 grams
Post Shredded Wheat – Original	1 cup has 0 grams
General Mills Cheerios – Original	1 cup has 1 gram
Arrowhead Mills – Sprouted Corn Flakes (gluten-free)	1 cup has 1 gram
Arrowhead Mills – Shredded Wheat (bite size)	1 cup has 2 grams
General Mills Kix – Original	1¼ cup has 3 grams

Cereals with Most Amounts of Sugar

The following brands of cereal have the *most* amounts of sugar:

Post Grape Nuts	1 cup has 10 grams
Kellogg's Fruit Loops	1 cup has 12 grams
General Mills Cocoa Puffs	1 cup has 12.5 grams
Cascadian Farms Granola	1 cup has 13 grams
General Mills Raisin Nut Bran	1 cup has 17.5 grams
Kellogg's Cracklin' Bran	1 cup has 17.5 grams
Back to Nature Sunflower & Pumpkin Seed Granola	1 cup has 22 grams
Back to Nature Sunflower & Pumpkin Seed Granola	1 cup has 22 grams
Udi's Gluten-Free Granola, Cherry Walnut	1 cup has 32 grams
Nature's Path, Fruit and Nut Granola, gluten-free	1 cup has 32 grams

Let's look at this. If four grams is one teaspoon, then 32 grams of sugar in one cup of cereal is 8 teaspoons of sugar! Can you even imagine putting that much sugar into your child's bowl of cereal?!

For a detailed list of sugar content in 1500 breakfast cereals, go to: http://www.ewg.org/research/childrens-cereals-sugar-pound/executive-summary.

Oatmeal

Plain oatmeal has less sugar than cereals:

Whole Foods 365 Instant hot oatmeal, multigrain with flax	1 packet has 0 grams
Bob's Red Mill Old Fashion Rolled Oats, whole grain	½ cup has 1 gram

Food Bars

Many people think food bars are easy and grab them for breakfast. These food bars (like cereal in a bar form) have the following amounts of sugar:

Nu Go - Slim– Raspberry Truffle Bar	1 bar has 2 grams
Cliff Bars	1 bar has 5 grams
Kind, Maple Pumpkin Seeds	1 bar has 6 grams
Earth's Best Sunny Days, strawberry	1 bar has 6 grams
Glutino, Apple, gluten-free	1 bar has 17 grams

Dairy-Free Beverages

Pouring milk on cereal can add an additional amount of sugar to the food, so purchase milk or milk alternatives that have no added sugar and are low in natural sugar. I use unsweetened vanilla alternative milk and add my own stevia or sweetener. By doing this, I control of the type and amount of sweetener in my milk. These dairy-free milks have the following amounts of sugar:

Pacific Brand unsweetened, vanilla hemp nondairy beverage
1 cup has 0 grams of sugar
Whole Foods 365 unsweetened, rice milk
1 cup has 0 grams of sugar
Dairy-free coconut milk, unsweetened
1 cup has 1 gram of sugar

Buying Bulk

Bulk foods can be a good way to purchase foods less expensively than packaged foods. Still, I was shocked to find high amounts of sugar in products I expected would be sold in raw and natural form. Even when buying bulk foods, read the labels well. Most of the fruits, granolas, crackers, and nuts have added sugar.

Most Important Meal of the Day

Breakfast is your most important meal of the day. When you wake up, your stomach is empty, so the food you take in will get absorbed like a sponge. Most importantly, it will give you energy and stamina for the day.

Make sure your breakfast takes care of you while it supports—and doesn't compromise—your family's health. Choose a breakfast that's low in sugar and high in nutrients with high-quality protein, fats, and carbohydrates. Then you'll take better care of your body, and your body will be able to take better care of *you*.

CHAPTER 8

Important Nutrients to Support Health

In today's modern world, it's hard to believe anyone could be deficient in nutrients. Yet statistics show that a high percentage of the U.S. population is either overweight or obese, only 10 percent eat a healthy diet, and 16 percent eat a poor diet.[64]

The President's Council on Fitness, Sports & Nutrition has said that eating habits have contributed to the obesity epidemic in the United States:

> About one third of U.S. adults (33.8%) are obese and approximately 17% (or 12.5 million) of children and adolescents aged 2–19 years are obese. Even for people at a healthy weight, a poor diet is associated with major health risks that can cause illness and even death. These include heart disease, hypertension (high blood pressure), type 2 diabetes, osteoporosis, and certain types of cancer. By making smart food choices, you can help protect yourself from these health problems.[65]

Part of the problem is the decline of nutrients in our food supply. According to Dr. Donald Davis of the University of Texas's Biochemical Institute:

> A recent study of 43 garden crops led by a University of Texas at Austin biochemist suggests that their nutrient value has declined in recent decades while farmers have been planting crops designed to improve other traits.

The study was designed to investigate the effects of modern agricultural methods on the nutrient content of foods. The researchers chose garden crops, mostly vegetables, but also melons and strawberries, for which nutritional data were available from both 1950 and 1999, and compared them both individually and as a group. [66]

As Davis said:

> We found that six out of thirteen nutrients showed apparently reliable declines between 1950 and 1999. These nutrients included protein, calcium, phosphorus, iron, riboflavin, and ascorbic acid. The declines, which ranged from 6 percent for protein to 38 percent for riboflavin, raise significant questions about how modern agriculture practices are affecting food crops.[67]

Two of the main reasons for the depletion of nutrients in our foods are that our soils are depleted and the topsoil has eroded. Most farmers aren't planting crops and tilling them under to nourish the soils and let them rest, as farmers used to do in the winter. Thus, the soils don't contain the nutrients they used to, resulting in food with lower nutrients. Good probiotics for the earth have been developed to improve farming, but I am not sure how many farmers are using these. (See Probiotics for the Garden, People, and Pets in the Resources section.)

Processing and cooking foods can also deplete the nutritional value of foods. What can we do about it? Sometimes we need to take high-quality supplements in order to prevent nutritional deficiencies.

All nutrients are important. We should make certain our children are getting all of the vitamins and minerals they need. You'll find a list of these and their exact requirements at the end of this chapter. Here are a few nutrients I think are important to mention specifically.

Iodine

Iodine is one of the most important nutrients supporting our health. It is an essential nutrient that supports the thyroid, our "master gland" which is central to all of our body's major functions.

The thyroid influences our metabolism, digestion, energy, body temperature, skin, hair, sleep, mental acuity, nervous system, sexual organs, and hormonal system. It would be very difficult to find a system that is *not* influenced by the thyroid. Because of the thyroid's widespread effects, its malfunction can significantly affect a person's life and be detrimental to long-term health. It is difficult to have a healthy thyroid without iodine.

What foods contain iodine? Soil is pretty much depleted of this nutrient, and there are few foods that contain iodine. Up until 1980, bakeries added iodine to bread. After 1980, they switched from adding iodine to adding potassium bromate. What does this mean? We have a certain amount of space for iodine in our thyroid gland. Our body can store about three months' worth of iodine in the cells. When we ingest potassium bromate, also called bromide, it acts like iodine and will take up the space in the thyroid reserved for iodine. It will *prevent* the body from absorbing the iodine it needs. The chlorine and fluoride that almost all municipal water companies in the United States add to water act the same way. These chemicals can all contribute to iodine deficiency.

Iodine is present in table salt. However, when it is exposed to oxygen, the iodine dissipates, so this is not really a reliable source. Also, table salt is actually refined sodium with added bicarbonates, chemicals, sugar, and preservatives. The minerals are removed, and the body interprets this table salt as toxic.

Real sea salt is full of minerals and nutrients our body needs. True sea salt is rich in electrolytes, which help our bodies absorb water and feed our body on a deep, cellular level. Most mineral salts have some iodine in them, in various amounts. Vitamin E and vitamin D are important nutrients that can help the body absorb iodine.

Vitamin E should be taken with an iodine supplement to help with iodine absorption.[68] Add some sunflower seeds to this mixture for a nutrient-dense composition. Foods rich in vitamin E are wheat germ, rice, oats, quinoa, broccoli, sprouts, spinach, dandelion greens, mint, almonds, and sunflower seeds.

The World Health Organization has said that iodine deficiency is the world's greatest single cause of preventable mental retardation. In addition, researchers at the University of Texas have reported their concern about iodine deficiency during pregnancy. One scientist claimed there's a likelihood of having subtle neurological deficiencies in babies born in the U.S. to mothers with iodine deficiencies. The same researchers have called on the U.S. government to boost America's iodine intake.[69]

Iodine Supplements

In his book *Iodine Why You Need It, Why You Can't Live Without It,* Dr. David Brownstein recommends an iodine supplement that contains both iodine and iodide. He states the thyroid needs both of them, with smaller amounts for children. Work with a health care professional who can provide proper testing, and follow your child's laboratory results.

Dr. Brownstein's book details how medical tests for iodine usually don't show the true picture of iodine deficiency. I recommend taking it with you to the doctor's office and having him do the iodine tests according to Dr. Brownstein's recommendations. One of Dr. Brownstein's ways of spotting a thyroid problem is a basal body temperature below normal, which is 97.8–98.2 degrees F. If your or your child's basal body temperature is consistently below 96.6 degrees F, that indicates a thyroid problem.

As a supplement for iodine, Dr. Brownstein recommends Lugol's Iodine and Iodoral Tablets, because both contain both iodine and iodide. The therapeutic actions of iodine are antibacterial, anticancer, antiparasitic, and antiviral. It elevates pH and is a mucolytic agent. The conditions he lists that can be therapeutically treated with iodine supplementation are: ADD/ADHD, atherosclerosis, breast diseases, fatigue, fibrocystic breasts, goiter, hemorrhoids, infections, hypertension, liver diseases, thyroid disorders, vaginal infections, sebaceous cysts, ovarian disease, prostate disorders, headaches and migraine headaches, and fatigue.

If you're concerned about idodine or the thyroid, If you're concerned about iodine or the thyroid, I highly recommend Dr. Brownstein's books I*odine: Why You Need It, Why You Can't Live Without It* and *Overcoming Thyroid Disorders*. His website is www.drbrownstein.com.

Magnesium

What is the percentage of Americans with inadequate intakes of magnesium from food based on estimated average requirements? Answer: 56 percent.[70]

Magnesium, a trace mineral, is necessary for hundreds of bodily functions. Magnesium deficiency has been linked to migraines, allergies, anxiety, asthma, attention deficit disorder, diabetes, calcification of soft tissue (including the heart valve), muscle cramps, osteoporosis, fibromyalgia, hearing loss, menstrual cramps, insomnia, irritability, trembling, and twitching.

Magnesium deficiency can also cause increased levels of adrenaline, which can create feelings of anxiety. A Brown University study found magnesium to be extremely beneficial for children with acute asthma. In addition, children with sensitive hearing may have low magnesium levels.[71]

Another factor for low magnesium may be the use of calcium supplements that don't contain magnesium. "High calcium intake can make magnesium deficiency worse," according to Forrest Nielsen.[72] He says additional magnesium can help. In an article on the USDA Agriculture Research Service website, Nielsen wrote, "The diets of many people do not contain enough magnesium for good health and sleep."[73]

Foods that contain magnesium are beans, whole grains, nuts, and vegetables—especially green, leafy vegetables. Some tasty magnesium-rich food choices for children are baked potatoes, bananas, coconut milk, peas, peanut butter, bean burritos, and cashews. Caffeine and alcohol can deplete magnesium. Caffeine-rich foods including coffee, tea, some energy drinks and bars, and various types of soda should be avoided.

Chromium and Sulfur

Chemical fertilizers used for growing non-organic foods destroy the natural sulfur and chromium in the soil. Therefore, foods grown in this way don't contain those nutrients. People who eat non-organically grown types of foods are more likely to have an insufficient amount of sulfur or chromium in their body.

Sulfur is a major nutrient we need in order to get oxygen into our cells. MSM is a natural form of organic sulfur. Sulfur is the third most prevalent element found in the body. Sulfur is one of the body's main nutrients and absolutely critical to our health. Without the proper levels of sulfur, our bodies aren't able to build healthy cells, and this leads to illness.

As noted earlier, although sulfur (MSM) is found in all organically grown foods, due to its unstable nature, it is quickly lost when food is processed, cooked, or stored. This is why a diet high in freshly picked, raw, unprocessed, whole, organic food is so vitally important to our diet.

One way you can get more natural sulfur into your body is to swim, bathe, or drink water from a natural spring or well that contains natural, organic sulfur. This type of water has been known for its healing qualities for centuries.

The powdered variety of sulfur (MSM) is 50 percent or more useless. Powdering it or combining it with magnesium sterate, which is used as filler in many supplements, can render the sulfur fairly useless.

The mineral chromium is important because it helps transport the glucose from the blood into the muscles. According to the National Institutes of Health, "Chromium is known to enhance the action of insulin, a hormone critical to the metabolism and storage of carbohydrate, fat, and protein in the body."[74] I believe chromium supplements have to be of a natural form, not synthetic. Synthetic forms of any vitamin can be harmful to the body.[75] [76] [77] Therefore, when buying supplements, look for whole, organic foods listed as the ingredients.

Berkeley Wellness Magazine noted that studies on vitamins are usually conducted with only synthetic forms of vitamins, not both synthetic and whole food. In my opinion, all studies should use both types to be complete and accurate.

CHAPTER 9

Vitamin D, the Sun, and Sun Protection

The sun promotes health and vitality. Still, we want to protect ourselves and our children from the sun during the summer. Which sunscreens are healthy to use? Not all are helpful, and many are harmful. Recent studies reveal that some sunscreens can cause vitamin D3 deficiency and increase the risk of skin cancer.[78]

Approximately 87 percent of the population is vitamin D deficient in the winter months. Seven out of 10 children and 70 percent of breastfed babies are deficient in vitamin D3, which affects their growth and development.[79] Because of these alarming numbers, many doctors recommend significant daily supplements of vitamin D and, more specifically, vitamin D3.

Vitamin D is a hormone known in its active form as calcitriol. A deficiency of calcitriol may be responsible for over seventeen cancers, autoimmune disease, multiple sclerosis, osteoarthritis, hypertension or high blood pressure, diabetes, depression, and genetic disorders, and may increase the risk of cardiovascular disease.[80] Rickets (bone softening) is a disease caused by vitamin D deficiency.

The American Medical Association recommends we get at least 15 minutes of direct midday sun, without applying sunscreen, several times a week. However, the American Academy of Dermatology says, "There is no scientifically validated, safe threshold level of UV exposure from the sun that allows for maximal vitamin D3 synthesis, without increasing skin cancer risk."[81] It is ultimately your decision, but avoid staying out in the sun and burning your skin due to prolonged exposure.

Humans have been getting their vitamin D from the sun for centuries, and foods with sufficient vitamin D are few.

Most experts agree with the American Medical Association's recommendations for sun exposure. The amount of skin exposed to sunshine correlates directly with how much vitamin D will be produced. The more skin exposed, the more vitamin D will be created. Also, people with darker skin need more sunlight than light-skinned people. We also need sunlight through our eyes without sunglasses each day.

The Danger of UVB Rays

For about 25 years, we have used sunscreens that block out UVB rays, but not UVA rays. UVB rays were thought to be the cause of skin cancer, but studies now reveal that sunscreens were blocking UVB cancer-protecting rays and allowing in UVA rays that can cause cancer. There is no vitamin D toxicity from sunshine, because UVA rays break down excess vitamin D. We can store vitamin D in fat cells and use it in the winter months if we get enough in the summer.

UVB rays are at their peak in the summer and are not available for most of the winter north of Atlanta, Georgia. When UVB rays stay on the skin's surface, they help the body make vitamin D3, which is why they were incorrectly blamed for causing skin cancer. The SPF rating only measured the UVB blocking power. Sunscreens reportedly reduce vitamin D3 levels in the blood by up to 99 percent.[82]

What do you do about sunscreen if you need to be outside for long periods? Stay in the shade when you can, wear protective clothing/ hats, and select the safest sunscreen you can.

Some sunscreens have carcinogenic ingredients and hormone disrupters that should be avoided: oxtinoxate, octisalate, oxybenzone, homosalate, avobenzone, and retinyl palmitate (a form of vitamin A). Check all sunscreens for these ingredients. They absorb easily through the skin and are toxic when combined with sun exposure.

Zinc oxide and titanium dioxide have been called safe, and reportedly do not penetrate the skin. But, my most recent research leads me to believe they are not safe. Micronized metals will penetrate the skin and enter the blood stream, resulting in cancer and tumors. Titanium dioxide (TiO_2) is a known carcinogen.

Dr. Elizabeth Plourde, in her research paper "Exposing the Hazards of Sunscreen," says there is concern that "sunscreen chemicals should be examined in relation to rising autism rates."[83] If you are interested in this subject, read her paper.

Which Sunscreens are Safe to Buy

Look for sunscreens that are non-nano, because extremely small particles can penetrate the skin. You want particles so large they cannot penetrate skin. The Environmental Workers Group (EWG) tested more than 1,500 sunscreens for safety and effectiveness. The sunscreens listed below contain either zinc oxide or titanium dioxide in some form. The ones listed with an asterisk are recommended as the safest.[84]

Thinkbaby and Thinksport **
UV Natural*
Soleo Organics*
Badger*
Loving Naturals*
Purple Prairie Botanicals*
Beyond Coastal
California Baby
Desert Essence
Episenical
Jason Natural Cosmetics
Estion
Caribbean Solutions
All Terrain

Kababa Skin Care
L'uvalla Certified Organic
Little Forest
Miessence
Trukid
Vanicream

Drinking carrot juice or eating carrots also gives the body some natural sun protection due to beta carotene.

CHAPTER 10

Recommended Nutritional Requirements

Nutrients are especially important for growing children because their organs and bones are still forming. The nutrient requirement charts below are from the Linus Pauling Institute for Micronutrient Research for Optimum Health.[85]

Micronutrient Needs of Children Ages 4 to 8 Years

For each micronutrient, the FNB sets a Recommended Daily Allowance or RDA for children ages 4 to 8 years. The table below lists the RDA for each micronutrient by gender.

Dietary Reference Intakes Set by the FNB:
RDA for Micronutrients During Childhood, Ages 4 to 8 Years

Micronutrient	*Males and Females*
Biotin	12 mcg/day (AI)
Folate	200 mcg/day[a]
Niacin	8 mg/day[b]
Pantothenic Acid	3 mg/day (AI)
Riboflavin	600 mcg/day
Thiamin	600 mcg/day
Vitamin A	400 mcg/day (1,333 IU/day)[c]
Vitamin B6	600 mcg/day
Vitamin B12	1.2 mcg/day
Vitamin C	25 mg/day
Vitamin D	15 mcg/day (600 IU/day)

Vitamin E	7 mg/day (10.5 IU/day)[d]
Vitamin K	55 mcg/day (AI)
Calcium	1,000 mg/day
Chromium	15 mcg/day (AI)
Copper	440 mcg/day
Fluoride	1 mg/day (AI)
Iodine	90 mcg/day
Iron	10 mg/day
Magnesium	130 mg/day
Manganese	1.5 mg/day (AI)
Molybdenum	22 mcg/day
Phosphorus	500 mg/day
Potassium	3,800 mg/day (AI)
Selenium	30 mcg/day
Sodium	1,200 mg/day (AI)
Zinc	5 mg/day
Choline[e]	250 mg/day (AI)
Alpha-Linolenic Acid[e]	900 mg/day (AI)
Linoleic Acid[e]	10 g/day (AI)

AI, adequate intake
[a]Dietary Folate Equivalents
[b]NE, niacin equivalent: 1 mg NE = 60 mg tryptophan = 1 mg niacin
[c]Retinol Activity Equivalents
[d]Alpha-tocopherol

[e]Considered an essential nutrient, although not strictly a micronutrient

Micronutrient Needs of Children Ages 9 to 13 Years

For each micronutrient, the FNB sets an RDA or AI for children ages 9 to 13 years. These recommendations are gender specific to account for the unique nutritional needs of boys and girls as they undergo puberty.

**Dietary Reference Intakes Set by the FNB:
RDA for Micronutrients During Childhood, Ages 9 to 13 Years**

Micronutrient	*Males*	*Females*
Biotin	20 mcg/day (AI)	20 mcg/day (AI)
Folate	300 mcg/day[a]	300 mcg/day[a]
Niacin	12 mg/day[b]	12 mg/day[b]
Pantothenic Acid	4 mg/day (AI)	4 mg/day (AI)
Riboflavin	900 mcg/day	900 mcg/day
Thiamin	900 mcg/day	900 mcg/day
Vitamin A	600 mcg/day (2,000 IU/day)[c]	600 mcg/day (2,000 IU/day)[c]
Vitamin B6	1 mg/day	1 mg/day
Vitamin B12	1.8 mcg/day	1.8 mcg/day
Vitamin C	45 mg/day	45 mg/day
Vitamin D	15 mcg/day (600 IU/day)	15 mcg/day (600 IU/day)
Vitamin E	11 mg/day (16.5 IU/day)[d]	11 mg/day (16.5 IU/day)[d]
Vitamin K	60 mcg/day (AI)	60 mcg/day (AI)
Calcium	1,300 mg/day	1,300 mg/day
Chromium	25 mcg/day (AI)	21 mcg/day (AI)
Copper	700 mcg/day	700 mcg/day
Fluoride	2 mg/day (AI)	2 mg/day (AI)
Iodine	120 mcg/day	120 mcg/day
Iron	8 mg/day	8 mg/day
Magnesium	240 mg/day	240 mg/day
Manganese	1.9 mg/day (AI)	1.6 mg/day (AI)
Molybdenum	34 mcg/day	34 mcg/day

Phosphorus	1,250 mg/day	1,250 mg/day
Potassium	4,500 mg/day (AI)	4,500 mg/day (AI)
Selenium	40 mcg/day	40 mcg/day
Sodium	1,500 mg/day (AI)	1,500 mg/day (AI)
Zinc	8 mg/day	8 mg/day
Cholinee	375 mg/day (AI)	375 mg/day (AI)
Alpha-Linolenic Acide	1,200 mg/day (AI)	1,000 mg/day (AI)
Linoleic Acide	12 g/day (AI)	10 g/day (AI)

AI, adequate intake
[a]Dietary Folate Equivalents
[b]NE, niacin equivalent: 1 mg NE = 60 mg tryptophan = 1 mg niacin
[c]Retinol Activity Equivalents
[d]Alpha-tocopherol
[e]Considered an essential nutrient, although not strictly a micronutrient

MSG: A Hidden Danger in Processed and Restaurant Foods

Monosodium glutamate (MSG) is categorized as an excitotoxin. According to Dr. Russell Blaylock, a neurosurgeon who wrote *Excitotoxins: The Taste that Kills,* these excitotoxins will stimulate and excite neurons in the brain to death, causing brain damage in varying degrees.

Today, MSG is frequently made by a fermenting process using starch, sugar beets, sugar cane, or molasses. MSG was discovered in 1908 by Japanese chemist Kikunae Ikeda. Professor Ikeda was trying to isolate a chemical in seaweed: kombu, a flavor enhancer. He came up with glutamic acid combined with a sodium molecule, which resulted in MSG. The component glutamate, or glutamic acid, is an excitatory amino acid neurotransmitter in the brain. These neurotransmitters in the brain are normal. But when there is an excess of them, they will be over-stimulated and die. This is extremely harmful to our brain health, according to Dr. Blaylock. Children and infants are even more vulnerable to this chemical.

When Professor Kikunae Ikeda founded the Ajinomoto Company and introduced his new product, it was a huge hit. MSG enhanced the flavor of food. It actually makes you think what you are eating tastes better because it works on the brain as a pleasure trigger. It can send pleasure impulses to the brain—until it kills that part of the brain. So, food that may normally taste a bit dull or bland may taste really great with MSG added to it.

The Japanese began using it in many foods, including the rations they gave to U.S. prisoners of war. The U.S. military became curious about why its soldiers loved the food rations they received as Japanese prisoners of war. After the presence of MSG was discovered in 1948, the military met with the largest food companies in the United States and discussed how MSG could be added to various food products.

MSG has since been added to a high percentage of processed foods and foods in almost all restaurants. Over the years, a greater amount of

MSG has been added to foods. The diet food industry has really benefited from MSG.

Still, Dr. Blaylock has tried for many years to educate people about these toxic additives in our food supply. (See his books listed in Resources.) As of 2010, the FDA had set no limit on how much MSG can be added to food. Some foods that contain MSG are NutraSweet and aspartame.

Theoretically, the long-term effects of MSG consumption can be attention deficit/hyperactivity disorder (ADHD), autism, and other learning disabilities. In adults, conditions such as Parkinson's, Alzheimer's, and Lou Gehrig's diseases, multiple sclerosis, auto-immune disease, sleep disorders, migraines, and the inability to lose weight may be linked to excitotoxin damage.

Hydrolyzed Proteins

Hydrolyzed proteins are flavor enhancers that have been chemically broken down into amino acids. As they're broken down during digestion, the resultant free glutamate joins with the body's free sodium to form MSG.

Free glutamate can cause the body to react as if a stimulating drug has been introduced into the nervous system. It can affect insulin metabolism and create excessive insulin secretion by the pancreas. Some common symptoms of this reaction are anxiety attacks, asthma-like symptoms, attention deficit disorder, burning sensations, and carpal tunnel syndrome. Additional disorders are chest pains, depression, diarrhea, disorientation and confusion, dizziness, drowsiness, and fatigue. Flushing, gastric distress, headaches and migraines, hyperactivity in children, infertility, and other endocrine problems may also occur. Insomnia, irregular or rapid heartbeat, joint pain, mood swings, mouth lesions, nausea and vomiting, numbness, seizures, shortness of breath, skin rash, slurred speech, stomachaches, tremors, and weakness may also develop.

Here is a partial list of hidden sources of MSG from *Excitotoxins:*

The Taste that Kills by Dr. Russell Blaylock. Some of the ingredients aren't MSG when they are originally added to food, but create MSG when they touch saliva. Many of these look like normal food ingredients. That is why buying whole, fresh foods and preparing your own food has become increasingly important for health.

Additives that always contain MSG:

- Monosodium glutamate
- Hydrolyzed vegetable protein
- Hydrolyzed protein
- Hydrolyzed plant protein
- Plant protein extract
- Yeast extract
- Textured protein
- Autolyzed yeast
- Hydrolyzed oat flour

Additives that frequently contain MSG:

- Malt flavoring and/or extract bouillon
- Broth
- Stock
- Flavoring
- Natural flavoring
- Seasoning
- Spices

Additives that may contain MSG or excitotoxins:

- Enzymes
- Soy protein concentrate or isolate
- Whey protein concentrate

Interestingly, no one requires these ingredients, which may contain MSG, to be listed on an ingredient label *as* MSG, even though MSG is listed when it's added in full form.

CHAPTER 11

What It Means to Eat Healthy

Many foods are not healthy foods. Packaged foods, fast foods, processed foods, bakery foods, restaurant foods, and some grocery store foods may contain refined grains, refined salt, refined sugars, trans fats, chemicals, and other extremely unhealthy ingredients. Just because a food is organic, gluten-free, vegetarian, or vegan does not necessarily mean that the food is healthy. Many labels list unfamiliar ingredients that leave you wondering what is *really* in the food. Many keep ingredients unknown. You may never know what is in a food or body care product. A product called "natural" may be entiely composed of chemically derived ingredients. That a product can be entirely composed of chemicals and still be labeled "natural" can be very misleading.

Carbohydrates

Many popular foods (including gluten-free) may be high in sugar and refined or processed flours (carbohydrates), which the body recognizes as sugar. In fact, many foods sold in "healthy" grocery stores, including baby foods and children's cereals and food bars, actually have huge amounts of added sugar and refined carbohydrates, which make them incredibly unhealthy. The body will register these nutrient-empty sugars and fiber-free carbohydrates as sugar, which then causes blood sugar to spike. This makes the body work hard to bring the blood sugar level into balance. When the body is constantly working to keep blood sugar regulated, it can become exhausted and unable to regulate it. This can result in diabetes.

For the body to process nutrient-empty (refined) food, it must pull nutrients from the body. This is one of the main reasons carbohydrates have a reputation for being unhealthy. It is not the carbohydrate that is unhealthy; it is the *type of* carbohydrate that is unhealthy. Carbohydrates are actually the body's preferred fuel.

Whole grains (teff, oat, millet, amaranth, buckwheat), seed flours (quinoa), bean flours (garbanzo bean, black bean), and nut flours (almond, coconut, walnut) that are nutrient and fiber dense are nourishing. They can provide your body with the fuel it needs.

I use sprouted, organic flour. (See Resources.) When I started making my recipes with healthier flours, they gained a richer flavor and higher protein content, and my children loved them.

Refined carbohydrates and unrefined carbohydrates are not converted into glucose in the same way. Unrefined carbohydrates (legumes, whole grains, vegetables) are rich in fiber and take longer to digest. This will not put additional pressure on the pancreas to produce insulin in an unhealthy way.

Refined carbohydrates (white refined flour, pasta, bakery goods) have little to no fiber. They convert to glucose quickly and put pressure on the pancreas to make insulin to get it under control. If too many of these refined carbohydrates are eaten on a continual basis, greatly increasing blood sugar levels, this will stress the pancreas, and eventually the body will have trouble making insulin. The body will turn its excess glucose into fat. This can result in excess weight and obesity.

A body with too much fat will also start ignoring the signal to take glucose from the blood. The blood sugar spikes from refined and empty food can also result in cravings. When the body is not getting the nutrients it needs, it will start begging for them.

Role of Fiber

When the body is provided with nutrient-dense food, it gets the nutrients it needs, and cravings should not result. I realized over the years how little fiber most people have in their diet. Diets high in healthy, naturally high-fiber foods are associated with healthy cholesterol, less risk of coronary heart disease, reduction in blood pressure, easier weight management, improved-blood sugar levels, reduced risks of certain types of cancer, better digestion, and healthier intestinal tracks.[86]

A healthy diet includes unprocessed, high-fiber foods such as peas, beans, vegetables, fruits, seeds, nuts, and whole grains. When looking at a package that says "whole wheat" or "whole grain" on the front, read the ingredient list and make sure it says "whole" before every grain listed. Ideally, gluten-free would be whole grain, seed, pea, or bean as well. But, watch out for gluten-free foods with large amounts of added sugar.

If a food is enriched or refined, it has had the nutrients and fiber removed. If the ingredient list contains only the name of the grain or seed, then it is *not* whole. Make sure all the grains (including rice) or seeds on the ingredient list are "whole."

The front of the package may indicate a product contains a certain ingredient, but then, when you look on the ingredient list, a totally different ingredient may be the major ingredient in the product. Although this is legal, it is very misleading. One pasta product I saw claimed to be gluten-free "quinoa pasta," but was mainly corn.

What Whole Grains Do You Look For?

Here is a list of whole grains: amaranth, whole grain brown rice, bulgur (cracked wheat), buckwheat, millet, oatmeal, popcorn, rolled oats, quinoa, sorghum, triticale, whole grain barley, whole grain cornmeal, whole rye, whole wheat, and wild rice.

The Nature of Gluten

More people these days are being diagnosed with gluten intolerance or celiac disease. Approximately 20 million Americans have gluten sensitivities. Gluten is a protein found in wheat, rye, spelt, and barley. "Technically, gluten refers to any of the more than 23,000 distinct proteins in wheat, and the term 'gluten related disorders' describes a wide spectrum of problems associated with its consumption."[87]

Because of hybridization, many grains that contain gluten today have 50–80 percent more gluten than they did one hundred years ago. The word *gluten* comes from the Latin word *glūten,* or glue. If you've ever made paper maché out of wheat flour and water, you can understand this mixture makes a glue. It can be very hard for the body to digest. Consuming gluten causes digestive issues, dandruff and skin disorders, kidney problems, and depression. Celiac disease is the most well-known condition linked to gluten intolerance, and it can be quite dangerous. Many people have told me they saw doctors and clinics for years without a proper diagnosis. It is commonly overlooked and misdiagnosed. Bloating and severe stomach pain after eating gluten is a good indication of gluten sensitivity.

Many people feel better when they eat a gluten-free diet. Those who have been diagnosed with conditions such as irritable bowel syndrome, leaky gut, eczema, and autism often find a reduction in symptoms when they consume healthier, gluten-free foods. If you have an enlarged stomach or experience digestive problems after eating a meal that includes gluten, consider avoiding gluten in any form.

Some gluten-free grain and flour alternatives are quinoa (a seed), coconut, teff, tapioca flour, gluten-free oats (labeled gluten-free), amaranth, buckwheat, corn, Job's Tears (or Hato Mugi), millet, montina (a wild Indian rice grass) rice, sorghum, wild rice, and bean flours such as garbanzo bean flour.

Tapioca is a starchy plant from the rain forest. Added to a free flour mixture, it will add a chewier, crustier consistency to the food. It can also make the food a little lighter in texture.

For a long time, oat flour was thought to contain gluten. But eventually, it was discovered that oat flour was stored in the same silos or transported in the same containers as wheat. So, truly gluten-free oats must be labeled gluten-free.

Teff is a Middle Eastern grain with high protein content while quinoa, a seed, is a complete protein food. It has more oil in the grain, so it has a chewier consistency than the other grains.

Alternatives to Wheat

I recommend eating gluten-free alternatives to wheat that are organically grown and whole grain. Foods grown with genetically modified seeds possibly contain the Bt-toxin. GMOs (genetically modified organisms) containing Bt toxin have the insecticide built right into the seed. It is in the tissues of the plant. A recent analysis shows Bt toxin, glyphosate, and other components of GMOs are linked to five conditions that may either initiate or exacerbate gluten-related disorders:

1. Intestinal permeability
2. Imbalanced gut bacteria
3. Immune activation and allergies
4. Impaired digestion
5. Damage to the intestinal wall

Gluten-related disorders are commonly accompanied by, and possibly triggered by, intestinal permeability, commonly called "leaky gut."[88] Leaky gut occurs when gaps form between intestinal cells, and large particles from the digestive tract enter the bloodstream, potentially triggering immune or allergic reactions.

The Bt toxin produced by genetically modified corn and soy kills insects by punching holes in their digestive tracts. A 2012 study confirmed that it punctures holes in human cells as well. Bt toxin is present in every kernel of Bt corn, survives human digestion, and has been detected in the blood of 93 percent of pregnant women tested and 80 percent of their unborn fetuses. This hole-punching toxin may be a critical piece of the puzzle in understanding gluten-related disorders.[89]

Even if you are not eating food containing the Bt toxin, you could be eating meat from an animal that ate food with Bt toxin. You might be getting it into your system through the meat. That's why eating certified, organic meats is highly recommended. Be a savvy consumer.

CHAPTER 12

Clean Water for Optimal Health

Water is a key nutrient to our health. Our bodies consist of 66–72 percent water. Water helps the blood transport oxygen, nutrients, and antibodies to all parts of the body. Many illnesses result from dehydration. When our bodies register that we are thirsty, we are already dehydrated. My children and I always drank a glass of pure mineralized water as soon as we woke up. When we wake up, our body is empty. Like a sponge, our bodies will readily absorb whatever we ingest. Therefore, a glass of high-quality, mineral-rich water will be utilized more efficiently. It is best not to drink liquids with meals. Doing so dilutes the digestive enzyme juices, making it harder to digest the food. It is best to drink between, not during, meals.

The Water Cure

Fereydoon Batmanghelidj, MD, studied water while he was a prisoner in an Iranian jail. There, he treated and cured about 3,000 prisoners using water and a little sea salt to treat what he called chronic intracellular dehydration. He found that most people are sick because of dehydration. After his release, he wrote many books on this subject.

The "water cure" that he prescribed is simply this: water. Drink an ounce of water for every two pounds of body weight daily. Someone weighing 200 pounds should drink 100 ounces of water a day. This is *in addition to* any other beverages.

Consume water first thing upon getting up in the morning, then drink it on a continual basis every two hours. Also put 1/8 teaspoon of sea salt on the tongue with every 16 ounces of water. This is a key component in the "water cure."

Also, put your water in glass containers. Some plastics can leach into the water. For children, you can find some glass water containers that are encased in rubber, with handles that makes them easy to hold and transport.

◆ ◆ ◆

Dr. Batmanghelidj recommended regular table salt, but I prefer to use unrefined sea salt that still has the minerals (electrolytes) in it. This is especially important for people suffering from allergies or asthma, because unrefined sea salt has an antihistamine effect.

There are different types of sea salt with different mineral content. Try a few different ones and see which you prefer. Celtic sea salt is supposed to be high in minerals. I like Bolivian Rose salt, too. (See Resources.) Try to buy a solar-dried salt or salt from mines. It may be cleaner and more nutrient-dense than most of what is available today. Mined salt comes from oceans that were less polluted in a time when the earth was richer in nutrients. That was before humans started strip mining and clear cutting, practicing poor farming methods, and dumping huge amounts of pesticides, fertilizers, and antibiotics into our water, soil, and air.

Chlorinated Water

Almost all public water supplies have added chemicals to the water supply, including sodium fluoride and chlorine, both of which are poisons. Chlorine was the first poison developed for warfare. Chlorine also destroys vitamin E in the body and beneficial probiotics in the intestines. "Industrial chemist J.P. Bercz, PhD, showed in 1992 that chlorinated water alters and destroys unsaturated essential fatty acids (EFAs), 14 of the building blocks of people's brains and central nervous systems."[90]

Dr. Champion-Olson, a board-certified naturopath and clinical nutritionist, told me that chlorine could destroy the probiotics in your system. It doesn't have to be straight tap water. A glass of tea made with chlorinated water can contribute to this destruction. *Probiotic* means "for life," which is appropriate because probiotics act as the major part of our immune system. This is only one good reason to avoid ingesting or absorbing chlorine into the body. Rebuilding the immune system's probiotics would be a good plan of action if you have to drink chlorinated water or take chlorinated showers, etc.

While showering or swimming in chlorinated water, the chlorine soaks into the skin cells. Our skin is our largest organ. That's why medicine is often given in a medicinal patch. Medicine can be absorbed through the skin directly into the bloodstream. Research linking swimming in chlorinated pools to cancer and other medical conditions continues to make headlines. The latest such studies come from the Centre for Research in Environmental Epidemiology in Barcelona, Spain. They indicate, among other things, that swimming in a pool with chlorine may damage lungs and increase the risk of developing cancer.[91]

Fluoride in the Water

Sodium fluoride and fluorosilicic acid are common chemicals added to our municipal water supply. The companies that produce aluminum and fertilizers generate a byproduct of sodium fluoride, which may also contain lead and arsenic. *Sodium* fluoride is the fluoride that the government adds to the water supply, under the pretext it is good for our teeth and health. However, dental studies conducted used *calcium* fluoride, which not the fluoride being added to the water supply.

According to Paul Connett, PhD, "Fluoride is a cumulative poison. On average, only 50 percent of the fluoride we ingest each day is excreted through the kidneys. The remainder accumulates in our bones, pineal gland, and other tissues. If the kidney is damaged, fluoride accumulation will increase, and with it, the likelihood of harm."[92] Fluoride affects the thyroid gland and all our enzymatic systems. Fluoride's side effects include weight problems, damage to our immune system, and other serious disorders. Chemically derived fluorides are completely different from naturally occurring fluorides.

Fluoride affects different people and people of various ages differently. According to Connett:

> The level of fluoride put into water (1 ppm) is up to 200 times higher than normally found in mothers' milk (0.005–0.01 ppm) (Ekstrand 1981; Institute of Medicine 1997). There are no benefits, only risks, for infants ingesting this heightened level of fluoride at such an early age (this is an age where susceptibility to environmental toxins is particularly high).[93]

Sweden, Denmark, Holland, Germany, Belgium, Norway, and France do not add fluoride to their water. Some of these countries have made it illegal to do so.

Posing a Question

Why is it we sometimes get an idea so ingrained in our minds it seems impossible to forget? One of those ideas for me was coconut oil. When I was growing up, I had been told coconut oil was bad because it contained cholesterol and saturated fat. As I started researching health and nutrition, I learned that pure organic coconut oil is actually good for us. In fact, it may be one of the best healing oils we can use for cooking and eating. It also moisturizes our skin.

The cholesterol in the coconut oil is the "good" cholesterol that helps balance the "bad" cholesterol. Because it supports brain health with its ketones, there is evidence it can help prevent Alzheimer's disease. I've had to change my mind completely about coconut oil.

So I pose another question: What if a doctor told you he wants to prescribe a drug that had not been approved by the FDA, making it illegal for him to prescribe it? What if he wanted your whole family to take it, but he wouldn't be able to regulate the amount each one of you received? What if it was not the drug the tests had shown to work? What if this drug had been proven *not* to work in the way he was prescribing? What if it also caused brittle bones in the elderly, cancer in boys, and severe thyroid problems, too? And, by the way, it was actually a toxic waste material. Would you take that drug?

I've become aware of the newest studies on this drug: fluoride. I grew up believing, as most people did, that fluoride was good for my dental health, that it would help prevent cavities. This is an idea so deeply ingrained into society's consciousness that it's hard to change the way we've been taught to think. However, my daughter lost one of her dearest friends in high school to a rare bone cancer. Why did this beloved boy suddenly develop such a terrible disease called osteosarcoma?

Recent Studies on Fluoride

Recently, I learned about a 2001 study on fluoride and osteosarcoma that took the form of a PhD dissertation at Harvard University. "The thesis, authored by Dr. Elise Bassin, found a strong, statistically significant relationship between fluoride exposure during the 6th through 8th years of life (the mid-childhood growth spurt) and the later development of osteosarcoma among young males."[94]

Dr. Bassin's findings show that "bone is the principal site for fluoride accumulation within the body, and the rate of accumulation is elevated during the periods of bone development. Thus the cells in the bone, particularly during the growth spurts, may be exposed to some of the highest fluoride concentrations in the body."[95] The findings also show that fluoride is toxic and carcinogenic. This rare form of cancer shows up in young men in their late teens and early twenties. Dr. Bassin's research and her findings have never been disproven.

I revisited the study conducted decades ago to promote fluoride as a way to prevent tooth decay. It was done in the cities of Newburgh and Kingston, New York, about 40 miles apart. They found:

> After 10 years of the trial (which was methodologically flawed), it looked as if there was a large decrease in dental caries in the fluoridated community, compared to the non-fluoridated community. However, when children were re-examined in these two cities in 1995 (50 years after the trial began), there was practically no difference in the dental decay in the two communities. If anything, the teeth in the non-fluoridated Kingston were slightly BETTER.[96]

The initial study measured no long-term effect, yet the use of fluoride in our water to provide better dental health was strongly promoted. Then as the long-term studies were done, they found fluoride did not help with dental health. In fact, adding it into the water supply caused other health problems. Fluoride was added in a way that was not regulated in dosage or concentration, and is likely causing a cumulative effect in people's bodies.

Of course, we need to have pure water to drink, but fluoride is not added to the water to purify the water. It is added with the idea that it helps prevent tooth decay. Interestingly, the studies on tooth decay used calcium fluoride, yet the fluoride added to drinking water is sodium fluoride and fluorosilicic acid. They can be contaminated with lead and arsenic, and are actually toxic waste from aluminum and fertilizer plants.[97]

Also, studies done by leading dental researchers show that the mechanisms of fluoride's benefits were mainly "topical not systemic." That means fluoride worked somewhat when put on the tooth topically, but it didn't work, if at all, when it was ingested from the water supply.[98, 99] My research tells me ingested fluoride can cause severe health problems, including but not limited to thyroid health problems,[100, 101, 102] brittle bones,[103] and cancer.[104,105]

Let me pose this question: if a toxic substance is found to *not* help and actually cause harm to the health of a populace, then why keep using it? Cities have spent a millions purchasing the toxic waste from fertilizer plants to put into civic water supplies. This is a "product" that has been proven to *not* be the correct type of fluoride, to *not* work in an ingested form, to cause osteosarcoma in males, and to *not* even help with dental health. It has not been approved as a drug, and its dosage cannot be regulated.

Studies show that dental decay has been *declining* in every country at about the same rate, even before fluoride was introduced. And it's still declining, whether communities have fluoride or not.[106 107] Is it because the toothbrush is more frequently used and our hygiene has improved?

I will forever wonder if my daughter's friend's death from osteosarcoma was a result of fluoride in our water supply. Fluoride has been added for so long and its value become so ingrained in our thoughts. But, it's time to free our water supply of this toxic waste, to keep our water clean and safe for the health of our citizens. It would be much more environmentally responsible to have a flouride-free public water supply, for our earth and our health.

Safe Water Supplies

Each year, water treatment facilities report a multitude of violations of the Safe Drinking Water Act. Many facilities have old, dirty water pipes transporting the water, including lead pipes. *New Scientist* reported a comprehensive survey of U.S. drinking water which revealed an array of hormonally active chemicals like MTBE (methyl tert-butyl ether), a chemical found in fuel and a potential human carcinogen in high doses, as well as atrazine, a U.S. pesticide banned in the European Union. Atrazine has been linked to reproductive problems in lab animals and is also linked to breast cancer and prostate cancer.

In 2010, *National Geographic* reported that drinking water in schools in 27 states was contaminated with toxic substances including lead.[108] In 2009, the Associated Press analyzed data from the EPA and found the public water in about 100 school districts contained lead, pesticides, and other toxins.[109] If this water is being pumped to schools, then it is also being pumped into homes and businesses.

Because toxins are currently in our water supply, put a water purification system in your house. You can absorb as many water-borne toxins through your skin in a shower or bath as you would by drinking eight glasses of water. At the very least, get a water purifier for your shower that removes chlorine and fluoride, and only use pure drinking water for cooking and drinking.

To water my vegetable and herb gardens with pure water, I bought a filter that takes out chlorine and other contaminants. The filter attaches directly to the garden hose. You can buy it in the RV/outdoor department at many stores for about twenty-five dollars, and it will last three to six months.

Reverse Osmosis

The reverse osmosis system works well for filtering water, but it also extracts the good minerals present in the water, as well as make the water acidic. If the water is void of minerals, your body will pull minerals/electrolytes from your system to process the water. Natural spring, well, or fresh water sources contain minerals/electrolytes and nutrients. When drinking purified bottled water, you can add some minerals/electrolytes (like a pinch of unrefined, high quality sea salt) to the water. When you do this, your body won't need to pull minerals from your body in order to process the water.

Bottled Waters

EPA standards for the Clean Water Act do not apply to bottled water. There is very little regulation on bottled water, which is why I recommend having your own filter. According to the Natural Resources Defense Council, the bottled waters with a higher pH and more nutrients were Fiji, Evian, San Pellegrino, Volvic, Trinity Springs, and Perrier. The Council also notes the reverse osmosis purified water by Coca Cola called Dasani has added magnesium (Epsom salts).[110]

What about vitamin waters? Many vitamin waters contain all kinds of ingredients like high-fructose corn syrup, artificial color, preservatives, and even caffeine. Make certain to read ingredient lists before you buy anything. Packaging can be very misleading.

Water Containers

The potentially hazardous chemical BPA is part of many plastic containers. Plastic containing BPA can leach it into the water; for example, when a water-filled plastic container is left sitting in a hot car. The plastic gets hot and leaches into the water. Plastic can have many negative effects on the body. If you buy plastic, buy plastics marked with #2, #4, or #5 on the bottom of the container. These are supposed to be safer. A stainless steel bottle is another good option. Do not use aluminum containers.

Infused Water

Water is so crucial to our health, but sometimes we just want something with a little more taste to it. Infusing water can be easy, inexpensive, nutritious, and delicious. When infusing water, make sure the fruits are cleaned completely with food-grade hydrogen peroxide, food-grade vinegar, or a really good vegetable wash—whether the fruit is organic or not.

Be cautious when using fruit slices from restaurants or bars. Studies and tests done on fruits and vegetables that are added to drinks in many of these establishments have tested high in bacteria and E. coli.

Mint is wonderful for fresh, infused water. It invigorates the mind, refreshes the senses, has antiseptic qualities, aids in digestion, helps with the function of the liver, and can help with fresh breath. There are quite a few different types of mint, and each has a wonderful, fresh quality. Mint is extremely easy to grow in a pot or garden, so you can grow mint year-round inexpensively and with little work. You can freeze purified water and mint in ice cube trays to keep on hand. These are nice for adding to teas, cool water drinks, cold soups, or sauces in the hot summer months. I give them to my dog, and it helps her have better dog breath!

Orange, lemon, lime, and grapefruit slices all add a little zing to water, as well as a bit of vitamin C. Lemon balm and other herbs that you may be particularly fond of are all healthful and fun to drink or use in recipes that call for water.

Infused water has very few calories and is a wonderfully healthy and fun way to enhance refreshing, hydrating water.

CHAPTER 13

Healthy Drink Choices

You can also hydrate with good, high-quality fruits and vegetables that are naturally high in water content. Cucumber, watermelon, celery, and carrots contain pure water rich in vitamins and minerals. Watermelon is 90 percent pure, clean water. When you have these real, whole fruits and vegetables as juices, you are receiving natural electrolytes as well as hydrating fluids. Fruit juices can be like drinking pure sugar, so I recommend (especially for children) having them eat the fruit in its whole form instead of drinking fruit juices. They can be extremely hydrating in their whole-food form. Coconut water is a good choice for an electrolyte-rich hydrating drink. It does contain natural sugar, so don't overdo it.

One last note about water: Masaru Emoto was born in Japan. He became known for his studies of water and its ability to change when "words of intent" (negative or positive) were applied to water in various forms. His work is fascinating and shows the environment of water directly affects its molecular structure. Mr. Emoto's book, *The Hidden Messages in Water,* contains photographs showing the molecular structure of the water before and after he applied words to the containers of water. As he played music, it affected the molecular structure of the water as well. The water crystal experiments consisted of exposing water to various words, pictures, or music, and then freezing and photographing the molecular structure of the crystals using microscopic photography.

Mr. Emoto claims there are many differences in the crystalline structure of the water, depending on the source of the water. The waters were taken from various places all over the world. A water sample taken from a pristine mountain showed a geometric shape when it was frozen. When polluted water was studied, the water showed very different water molecules. One of his first experiments with photographing water molecular structure was intriguing. He put water from the same exact source in identical plastic jugs and left them overnight with labels of words or sayings on them. The molecular structure of the water in the jugs with negative sayings changed and looked like pus. On the other hand, the molecular structure of the water in the jugs with positive words attached—words like love and gratitude—looked absolutely beautiful, like snowflakes. The comparison was startling. You can see his photographs at http://www.masaru-emoto.net/english/index.html.

Given that words affect the water in jugs, shouldn't this cause us to ponder the effects of negative talk or negative self-talk? What does negative thought do to the water in our body or the water around us in our life? It's food/water for thought.

Juices and Juicing

When we juice foods, we get the nutrient density without the fiber. This makes it less work for the body to absorb. This is extremely beneficial for someone who needs intense nutrition and isn't able to consume whole food or hardly any food. We can get intense nutrients with living enzymes to feed our cells on a deep cellular level when juicing. Fresh juice alkalizes us and flushes out the toxins in our cells. The highly antioxidant-rich nutrients are an amazing way to cleanse the body of toxins. A juice cleanse can be a great way to boost your energy, balance your blood sugar, brighten your skin, and rejuvenate your hormones. I love to juice wheatgrass and barley grass, sunflower sprouts, and various other chlorophyll-rich foods.

Nutrients start to disperse after about 20 minutes, so drink the juice immediately. "Vegetable juice is HIGHLY perishable so it's best to drink all of your juice immediately," according to Dr. Joseph Mercola.[111] When buying fresh juice, make sure the juice is made for you right then, not earlier that day or the night before.

It is amazing how full you can feel after drinking a large glass of vegetable or fruit juice. I try to juice at least once a day. I usually have at least three carrots, cucumber, and celery in my juice. When I am cutting vegetables, I save the pieces I don't use for my next juicing (the end of the celery, the rind of the watermelon, the base of the lettuce, the stalks of the broccoli). I juice almost all of the skins. About the only skins I don't juice are melons like cantaloupe, because they are prone to mildew. The rinds of fruits like watermelon and citrus fruits are incredibly antioxidant packed. You can juice them, but they taste strong. I have juiced whole lemons when I am juicing a good bunch of heavy greens. The lemons give your fresh juices with lots of greens a kick and take out some of the heavy green taste. I also add a pinch of sea salt to my fresh juices. It makes it taste better and adds some nutrients that help the body optimally absorb nutrients, like potassium. I always make sure I have cleaned my fruits well, especially if I am juicing the skin.

Juicing can be an excellent way of fasting. You can get great nutrient density without all of the calories. This is also a good way to diet, without the intense hunger pangs. Just juice, juice, juice for life!

Wheatgrass Juice

Wheatgrass is a unique and beneficial food to juice. Dr. Yoshihide Hagiwara, president of the Hagiwara Institute of Health in Japan, advocates the use of grass as food and medicine because it is rich in chlorophyll. Chlorophyll is similar to hemoglobin, a compound in blood that carries oxygen. According to Ann Wigmore in her book *The Wheatgrass Book,* regularly drinking freshly juiced wheatgrass:

- Increases red blood cell count and lowers blood pressure.
- Cleanses the blood, organs, and gastrointestinal tract of debris.
- Stimulates metabolism and the body's enzyme systems by enriching the blood.
- Aids in reducing blood pressure by dilating the blood pathways throughout the body.

- Stimulates the thyroid gland, correcting obesity, indigestion, and a host of other complaints.
- Restores alkalinity to the blood. The juice's abundance of alkaline minerals helps reduce over-acidity in the blood.
- Can be used to relieve many internal pains and has been used successfully to treat peptic ulcers, ulcerative colitis, constipation, diarrhea, and other complaints of the gastrointestinal tract.
- Is a powerful detoxifier, and liver and blood protector. The enzymes and amino acids found in wheatgrass can protect us from carcinogens like no other food or medicine.
- Strengthens our cells, and chemically neutralizes environmental pollutants and toxic substances like cadmium, nicotine, strontium, mercury, and polyvinyl chloride.
- Offers the benefits of a liquid oxygen transfusion since the juice contains liquid oxygen.

Oxygen is vital to many body processes. It stimulates digestion (the oxidation of food), promotes clearer thinking (the brain utilizes 25 percent of the body's oxygen supply), and protects the blood against anaerobic bacteria. Cancer cells cannot exist in the presence of oxygen.[112] Recent studies show that wheatgrass juice has a powerful ability to fight tumors without the usual toxicity of drugs that also inhibit cell-destroying agents. The many active compounds found in wheatgrass juice cleanse the blood, and neutralize and digest toxins in our cells.

Dr. Bernard Jensen, a renowned nutritionist, wrote *Health Magic Through Chlorophyll from Living Plant Life* in which he mentions several cases where his patients' red blood cell count doubled in a matter of days just by soaking in a chlorophyll-rich bath. He also says that blood builds more quickly when the person drinks chlorophyll-rich fresh juices on a regular basis.[113]

Juicers You Can Use

There are some really good juicers on the market. A juicer is an investment, but it will give you really dense nutrients that are so beneficial to health. I think the hand-turn wheatgrass juicer is the best choice. It is less expensive and more reliable. Large juicers usually don't juice grasses. Grass juicers don't handle large vegetables very well. You really need to have two different types of juicers: one for the grasses, and one for large fruits and vegetables. (Check Appendix B for types of juicers.)

Juice Fasts and Feasts

Juicing is great for everyone. For people who are trying to heal from various diseases, it can be especially powerful due to its nutrient-rich, antioxidant enzymes. In an article titled "All About Insulin," Nina Nazor wrote, "Insulin is a hormone secreted by your pancreas, and its function is to regulate blood glucose levels. Insulin works like a key to open the door of the cells so glucose—the fuel you get from food—can come inside and be converted into energy."[114] For diabetics, the following foods have an insulin type of action: asparagus, avocados, bitter melon, black pepper, Brussels sprouts, carrots, cinnamon, cucumbers, fennel, garlic, ginger, grapefruit, guava, parsnips, raw green vegetables, onions, leeks, sweet potatoes, tomatoes, winter squash, wheatgrass, sprouts, and yams.

These are good choices for diabetics—or anyone, really. Just pick a few and vary them with the seasons as often as you can. At the Tree of Life, where I studied raw food and organic gardening, they did not put carrots in the juices for diabetics because of the higher sugar content of the vegetable. Keep this in mind if you are diabetic. Gabriel Cousens, MD, who wrote *There Is a Cure for Diabetes,* promotes juicing. In his book, he talks about juice "feasting." When I am drinking these fresh, nutrient-dense juices, I never feel hungry or tired.

For people with O blood types, which are known as protein types, Dr. Mercola said:

> If you are a protein type, juicing needs to be done cautiously. Celery, spinach, asparagus, string beans, and cauliflower would be your best vegetables to juice. You can add some dark, leafy greens like collards, kale, and dandelion greens, but do so cautiously and pay careful attention to how you feel.[115]

You may also want to initially limit your serving size of juice to no more than 6 oz., and store it properly and drink smaller amounts throughout the day.

To make drinking vegetable juice compatible with protein type metabolisms which need large amounts of fat, it is important to blend a source of raw fat into the juice. Raw flax seed oil, raw hemp seed oil, avocado, coconut oil, or freshly ground flax seed are the sources of raw fat I most recommend. In addition to adding a source of raw fat to your juice, you may also find that adding some, or even all, of the vegetable pulp into your juice makes it more satisfying.

Interestingly, I had been adding about a tablespoon of pulp back into my juice even before reading this information. I also add about a teaspoon of hemp oil, chia seeds, flax seed oil, or coconut oil to my smoothies and juices. I had been listening to my body and knew what it needed, even before I knew why. Listen to your body, and find out what works best for you.

Powerhouse Ingredients

Greens are a powerhouse of nutrients. They contain potassium, phosphorus, calcium, magnesium, iron, and zinc, along with vitamins A, C, E, and K. They have folic acid, chlorophyll, and micronutrients. Are you thinking, "Oh my goodness, greens for breakfast?" Yes! They are full of fiber. In traditional Asian medicine, the color green is related to the liver, emotional stability, and creativity. Greens aid in purifying the blood, strengthening the immune system, and improving liver, gall bladder, and kidney function. The nutrients in greens can help fight depression, clear congestion, and improve circulation, which can help keep skin clear and blemish-free.

Celery is a natural electrolyte and is hydrating. Carrots are a good blood regulator, and beneficial to people who have eye problems. Cucumbers, which are full of nutrients and natural electrolytes, are great for nourishing the skin. Watermelon is a great diuretic. Kale is known as the king of greens. When writing about kale and its benefits, Diane Dyer, MS, RD, points to the high content of calcium, vitamin C, vitamin B6, folic acid, vitamin A in the form of beta-carotene, vitamin K, potassium, manganese, copper, and even the plant form of omega-3 fatty acids (alpha-linolenic acid). In addition to the carotenoid beta-carotene, kale contains other very important carotenoid molecules called lutein and zeaxanthin, both necessary for eye health, and too many more to list, with even more yet to be identified.[116]

Just a note about sea salt and potassium: Jim Bolen wrote in his paper "Histamine/Anti-histamine and the Dangers of Taking Anti-histamine," "A person needs 1/8 teaspoon salt (3/4 gram) for every 8 ounces (250 cc) orange juice for the potassium to be used by the cells in the body."[117] Organic juice is loaded with potassium that our bodies cannot use without salt. Thus, when a person drinks orange juice and does not take enough salt to allow the potassium to enter human cells, histamine is released to take care of the problem. When histamine is released, symptoms like hay fever, itching, nausea, vomiting, and sleep disorders can occur. But when potassium is properly absorbed, it provides the body with a natural antihistamine that combats histamine symptoms.

Dr. Batmanghelidj, mentor to Jim Bolen, explains this clearly in his books. In *ABC of Asthma, Allergies and Lupus*, he notes that adding salt to orange juice balances the actions of sodium and potassium in maintaining the required volume of water inside and outside the cells. In some cultures, salt is added to melon and other fruits to accentuate their sweetness. These fruits contain mostly potassium. By adding unrefined sea salt to them before eating, a balance between the intake of sodium and potassium results. The same could be done to other fruits.[118]

Some foods need to be lightly steamed before being eaten because they contain phytic acid, which acts like an antinutrient, so they may not be good choices for juicing. (The phytic acid will reduce the absorption of valuable minerals such as calcium, magnesium, and zinc.) Foods containing phytic acid are blackberries, broccoli, cauliflower, carrots, figs, and strawberries. The vegetables must be lightly steamed or cooked to help neutralize the phytic acid.[119] The five goitrogenous chemicals in broccoli can disrupt the body's ability to use iodine. This can be a problem if someone has a thyroid deficiency or low iodine.[120]

Tomatoes are best when vine-ripened. If tomatoes are green-picked and later ripened, they can weaken the kidney–adrenal function.[121] Spinach, beet greens, and chard are high in oxalic acid. These particular greens should be "taken in limited quantities by those with mineral deficiencies or loose stools because of the laxative effect and the calcium-depleting effect of their substantial oxalic acid content."[122] Oxalic acid binds with calcium. If there isn't a good source of calcium in your food, the body will pull it from the bones to bind with the oxalic acid. This can harm your kidneys. The oxalic acid can also affect the absorption of iron. When eating spinach, have some vitamin C–rich food with it to help the body absorb the iron in the spinach more efficiently.

I like to add a little coconut water, kefir, or kombucha to my drinks as an added benefit for my immune system. To support your immune system, you can add the probiotics or fermented drinks with their beneficial flora. Drink this in the morning when your stomach is empty and has the ability to absorb it more readily.

CHAPTER 14

Recipes for Healthy Drinks

Where I grew up, tea parties with children were a tradition. I fondly remember hosting tea parties when I was a young girl. My parents loved to drink tea, so I grew up drinking it in the mornings or late in the afternoon. Even today, when my daughter is home, one of our favorite things to do is watch movies, play backgammon, and drink tea.

Legend has it that tea was discovered by Chinese emperor Shen Nung in 2737 BC. His servant was boiling water under a tree and some leaves blew into the water. Shen Nung, a renowned herbalist, decided to try the infusion, and this resulted in what we now call tea. Tea is hot water that is infused. Dried leaves or flowers are commonly packaged these days as tea.

Making tea is easy. Place one teaspoon of dried tea or one tea bag in a teapot or tea cup, add a cup or two of hot water, and steep for two to five minutes. The hot water for green teas should be 140 degrees F. You don't want to use water that is too hot, because it can harm the tea enzymes. Drink it plain, or add a drop or two of stevia, xylitol, or honey to sweeten. You can also add a sprig of mint or squeeze some fresh lemon juice for added flavor.

Teas

TULSI TEA

Tea is a great way to hydrate and reap the benefits of various healing and soothing herbs. Years ago when I was working on our book *Alive and Cooking* with my friend and co-author Maryann De Leo, she stayed at my home and brought tulsi tea with her. We drank a variety of absolutely delicious tulsi teas for a week.

I love this tea that's been used by the Ayurvedic practice for centuries and documented as far back as 5000 BC. In fact, tulsi tea is at the heart of India's Ayurvedic holistic health practice. In India, the sacred tulsi plant is known for promoting a healthier respiratory system and better vision as well as reducing stress. Dr. Singh, author of *Tulsi: Mother Medicines of Nature,* wrote that tulsi is one of the best stress adaptogens. That means it can help you relax and stay calm, and can boost your system to handle stress better. So, when it starts getting too wild around the house, everyone can sit down with a cup of tulsi tea and relax.

Overall, Tulsi is said to balance the health of the digestive system, promote a healthy metabolism, support skeletal and joint support, assist in normalizing cholesterol levels, boost stamina, help with mucus problems, and protect against free radicals. It comes in a variety of flavors. I served one of my tulsi teas to a 58-year-old client one day. About an hour after he left, he called me and asked, "What was that drink you gave me? I feel like Superman!" I told him, "Tulsi tea." He went out and bought different varieties and now drinks it almost every day.

GINGER TEA

Ginger tea, one of my favorite teas for the immune, digestive, and circulatory systems, can be especially good for aiding digestion. It's great to sip it if you have a queasy stomach. You can find ginger root at the grocery store, usually by the root vegetables or mushrooms. The skin should be smooth and tight, not wrinkly, and the root firm. Ginger root is available in all different sizes. Keep it in a cool, dry, dark place.

Ingredients:

1-inch piece fresh ginger root
2 c. or more of hot water
1 drops of liquid stevia to sweeten (optional)

Directions:

1. Grate or thinly slice ginger root.
2. Pour warm or hot (not boiling) water over it and steep about 5 to 20 minutes.
3. Strain.
4. Add a few drops stevia or honey for sweetness, if desired.

TURMERIC "TEA"

This tea would be for older children. Turmeric is a wonderful spice for restorative properties, including anti-inflammatory, antioxidant, and antimicrobial properties. It is a great blood purifier, and it helps hydrate dry skin. My daughter Amanda came home one day from college and said she had been adding ½ teaspoon to a cup of warm (not boiling) water and drinking it as a tea. (It is not an "official" tea, but that is what we call it.) She made me some, and I've been drinking it ever since!

In fact, what I do is I make this tea and drink it while I am letting my other tea steep, then I drink my other tea.

Juice Recipes

All of these juice recipes are vegan, vegetarian, raw, and gluten-free. You can add a pinch of unrefined sea salt to these juices for added electrolytes. When I make a green drink or juice, I sometimes will add a tiny bit of wheat or barley grass to my mixture for the added health benefits. It is a strong taste, but a tiny bit (a blade or two) usually doesn't make too much of a difference in the taste.

You can strain these drinks if they are made in a blender, but the fiber is healthy. I would suggest you keep it in the drink.

PEAR AND APPLE JUICE WITH GREENS

Ingredients:

2 cups or ¼ head of romaine lettuce

1 apple (with the skins on and the stem and seeds removed)

1 pear (with the skins on and the stem and seeds removed)

⅛ tsp. whole sea salt

Directions:

1. Juice the lettuce and apple and pear in a juicer.
2. Add the sea salt.
3. Drink at room temperature within 20 minutes if possible.

Serves one.

CARROT JUICE

Carrot juice is great for the eyes and can also provide the body with natural sun protection.

Ingredients:

4-5 whole, clean carrots

Directions:

Juice carrots and serve immediately.

Juice 4 large carrots per person.

CELERY AND CUCUMBER JUICE

Ingredients:

2 stalks of celery

¼- ½ of a cucumber

Optional: pinch of sea salt

Directions:

Juice all ingredients and serve immediately. Serves one.

CELERY, CARROT, AND CUCUMBER JUICE

Ingredients:

2 stalk of celery

¼–½ of a cucumber

2 carrots

Optional: pinch of sea salt

Directions:

Juice all ingredients and serve immediately.

Serves one.

LIME/LEMONADE FOR CHILDREN (more than 1 year of age)

Ingredients:

Juice of one whole, organic lime or lemon with about 1 Tablespoon of the clean skin of the fruit (juiced).

1½ c. pure, non-chlorinated water

A few drops to ½ a dropper of liquid stevia

Pinch of unrefined, high quality sea salt

Directions:

1. Juice the lemon or lime and add it to the water.
2. Add stevia and stir.
3. Serve at either room temperature or cool.
4. A warm lemon drink is soothing in the winter as well.

Note: This makes a good popsicle if you pour it into a popsicle mold and freeze. Variation: Add a few leaves of kale or romaine lettuce to this mixture and juice it.

Serves one.

BASIC GREEN DRINK

Ingredients:

1 c. fresh leafy greens

½ cucumber

Juice of half a lemon (optional - with the skin).

1 or 2 dates (non-sulfured), pitted and soaked in water for an hour

½ an avocado (pitted and peeled)

Pinch of unrefined sea salt

2 c. non-chlorinated water

Variation:

Substitute lime juice for lemon.

Directions:

1. Place all ingredients in a powerful blender and blend. Add more water if the drink is too thick.
2. Drink this within 20 minutes of making.

Notes:

Greens can be romaine lettuce, baby spinach, baby kale, green leaf lettuce, or a combination of any of these. Kale is an excellent choice.

Variations:

1. Substitute a cored apple or pear for the dates.

Serves one.

INFUSED WATER

Ingredients:

3 c. high-quality, non-chlorinated water

¼ c. orange slices, cucumber slices or a few springs of fresh mint

Directions:

1. Combine all ingredients.
2. Let set for an hour or more.
3. Drain leaves or fruit out of the water, leaving only the water.

Notes:

1. This recipe is easy to double or triple.
2. Consume at room temperature or refrigerate to enjoy a cooler beverage.

Serves two.

Drink Recipes

FRUITY COCONUT DRINK

Ingredients:

1 c. fresh organic fruit of choice (fresh berries are a good choice)

1 T. fresh organic sprouts (broccoli or sunflower seed is a good choice)

1½ c. organic, unsweetened vanilla coconut milk

4 drops of stevia liquid or 1 medjool date (pitted and soaked until soft)

Directions:

1. Place all the ingredients in a blender, blend until smooth.
2. Drink at room temperature or refrigerate to drink later.

Note:

Suggestions for fruit: strawberries, blueberries, cherries, raspberries, blackberries, huckleberries, and peaches. Frozen is fine, but fresh is best!

Serves one.

FRUITY COCONUT, PROTEIN POWER SMOOTHIE

Ingredients:

1 c. fresh, organic fruit of choice (freshly pitted cherries or blueberries are good)

½ or 1 banana

½- 1 T. raw, organic sunflower seed sprouts (any sprout such as broccoli sprouts, snow pea sprouts, radish sprouts would work well)

1½ c. unsweetened vanilla, organic coconut milk

2 T. Vanilla, Protein Powder (I use Garden of Life brand)

½ tsp. cold pressed, organic flax or hemp seed oil
1 tsp. organic, pure, coconut oil
2 dates, pitted and softened by soaking them in a little water for about 20 -30 minutes.
¼ tsp. fresh, soft bee pollen (optional)
Note: Add more coconut milk or a little of the date water if it is too thick.

Directions:

Place all ingredients in a blender and blend until smooth.
Drink at room temperature immediately.

Variation:

1. Substitute a few drops of stevia or a ½ tsp. of xylitol for the dates.
2. You can add more protein powder, if your child is older.

Serves one.

Note:

Fresh bee pollen is rich in protein, vitamins, minerals, beneficial fatty acids, carotenoids, and bioflavonoids. These are antiviral and antibacterial. They help in lowering cholesterol as well as stabilizing and strengthening capillaries. It is the only plant source that contains vitamin B12. If the pollen is fresh, it delivers at least 20 amino acids, the building blocks of protein required to build all the cells in the body including blood, skin, organs, and bones.

YUMMY POWER SMOOTHIE

This was one of my children's favorite smoothies. Serves One.

Ingredients:

1½–2 c. of unsweetened, organic almond, rice or coconut milk

2 T. pure, raw, organic, sprouted apricot, sunflower or almond seed butter

1 banana

2–3 heaping T. Garden of Life Protein Powder (vanilla)

3 drops of stevia or a couple of softened and pitted dates

1 tsp. pure, cold pressed, organic flax or hemp seed oil

1 tsp. pure, extra-virgin, organic coconut oil

Pinch of sea salt

Directions:

1. Place all ingredients in a blender and blend until creamy. (You can add more protein powder if your child is used to this drink or if they are older.)
2. Drink at room temperature.

Variation:

1. Add a 1cup of pitted cherries or blueberries to this for added vitamin C.
2. Add fresh bee pollen. See **Fruity Coconut, Protein Power Smoothie** for a description of its benefits.
3. Add half a pitted, peeled avocado to the smoothie.

Note:

1. Soften dates by soaking them in a little water.
2. You can add more protein powder, if your child is older.
3. You can buy raw, organic, sprouted nut and seed butter from Blue Mountain Organics.

BREAKFAST SMOOTHIE

Ingredients:

½ c. vanilla, unsweetened organic coconut yogurt

1½ c. unsweetened, organic, vanilla coconut milk

1 c. pitted organic cherries or berries (frozen work, but fresh is better)

2 T. pure, raw, organic, sprouted apricot or pumpkin seed butter

¼ tsp. ground Ceylon cinnamon

1 banana

2–4 T. protein powder (I use Garden of Life vanilla or hemp seed protein)

1 tsp. organic, cold pressed hemp or flax seed oil

1 T. pure, virgin, organic coconut oil

Directions:

Blend until smooth. Add more milk if it is too thick.

Variations:

1. Add 2 T. of cooked organic quinoa.
2. For a sweeter version, add ½ tsp. of xylitol or a few drops of stevia liquid to the blender with the berries. I use the toffee, vanilla, or berry-flavored Sweet Leaf brand stevia.
3. Add ½ an pitted, peeled avocado.
4. Add a tsp. of maca root powder.
5. You can buy raw, organic, sprouted nut and seed butter from Blue Mountain Organics.

Serves one.

YUMMY MANGO SMOOTHIE

Ingredients:

2 organic mangos peeled, seeded and cut into chunks.

½ c. organic baby, spinach, romaine lettuce, baby kale or baby swiss chard

1 c. pure water

½ tsp. organic cold-pressed hemp or flax seed oil

1 tsp. pure, organic coconut oil

Pinch of unrefined sea salt

Directions:

1. Place all ingredients in a blender and blend until smooth.
2. Add water if it is too thick.
3. Serve immediately.

Variations:

1. Add ½ an pitted, peeled avocado.
2. Add a tsp. of maca root powder.

Serves one.

Non-Dairy Milks

MILK WITH PIZAZZ!

Ingredients:

1 c. organic coconut milk (fresh, unsweetened, vanilla is good)
1 organic carrot juiced
½ organic beet juiced
1 medjool date, pitted and soaked in a little water for 20 minutes (optional)

Directions:

1. Blend in a blender.
2. Enjoy at room temperature or refrigerate for later.

Serves one.

NON DAIRY NUT MILK

Ingredients:

1 c. of your organic nut of choice
3 c. of filtered or spring, mineral rich water
¼ tsp. xylitol or a few drops of stevia to taste
⅛ tsp. unrefined, sea salt

Directions:

1. Soak nuts and/or seeds for 18 hours in enough non-chlorinated warm water to cover them by an inch. After 18 hours, drain off the water.
2. Blend the 3 cups of new, fresh, non-chlorinated water and nuts in a blender until smooth.
3. Strain through a nut bag cloth.
4. Add the xylitol or stevia and blend until smooth.

5. Drink immediately at room temperature or refrigerate for later.

Certain stevia brands come in flavors. I use the Sweet Leaf toffee flavor for my nut milks.

Note: You can use pine nuts, walnuts, sunflower seeds, almonds, or a combination of the some or all of these. If you buy sprouted, raw seeds or nuts, you won't need to soak them to remove the phytic acid. They will already be phytic acid free, if sprouted.

Serves one to two.

◆ ◆ ◆

I started experimenting with alternative milks because I couldn't find ones in the supermarket that were organic and/or not filled with sugar. This rice milk has become one of my absolute favorites. I do sometimes use pre-cooked rice, but freshly cooked rice is best.

RICE MILK

Ingredients:

1 vanilla bean

1 c. whole-grain, organic rice (freshly cooked)

2 c. non-chlorinated water

Stevia to taste (a couple of drops)

Dash of sea salt

Directions:

1. Split vanilla bean and use a sharp knife to scrape out the inside of the bean. Put scrapings in a blender.
2. Combine all ingredients in a blender and blend well.
3. Strain through a nut milk bag, or simply drink it as a thicker version. (The more rice you add, the thicker the milk will be.)

Variations:

1. You can omit or use an alternative vanilla flavor for this milk. Toffee or vanilla flavored stevia (by Sweet Leaf) is one I sometimes use instead of the vanilla bean. Pure vanilla extract is another choice.
2. You can add a soaked date for sweetening.

Serves one to two.

QUINOA MILK

Ingredients:

1 vanilla bean or ½ tsp. vanilla extract
1 c. organic, whole (freshly-cooked) quinoa
2 c. non-chlorinated water
Stevia to taste (optional)
Dash of sea salt

Directions:

1. Split vanilla bean and use a sharp knife to scrape out the inside of the bean. Put scrapings in a blender.
2. Combine all ingredients in a blender and blend well.
3. Strain through a nut milk bag, or simply drink it as a thicker version. (The more quinoa you add, the thicker the milk will be.)

Notes:

1. You can omit or use an alternative vanilla flavor for this milk. Toffee or vanilla-flavored stevia (by Sweet Leaf) is one I sometimes use instead of the vanilla bean.
2. You can add a soaked date for sweetening.

Serves one.

I use almond milk for many things, including as the liquid in my smoothies. I make my milk without sweetener and then add what I need to make it sweeter, depending on what I am using it for. I like to add a few drops of stevia most of the time. To flavor nut milks for drinking or to use on granola, I like to use the toffee stevia drops by Sweat Leaf. If I am using it for a recipe, I use plain stevia. My friend Maryann, who co-authored the book *Alive and Cooking* with me, likes vanilla-flavored stevia. It is just a matter of personal opinion. Find out what your favorite is!

ALMOND MILK

Ingredients:

1 c. organic almonds

¼ tsp. organic, unpasteurized apple cider vinegar (optional for soaking the nuts to remove phytic acid)

3 c. non-chlorinated water

¼–½ dropper of liquid stevia (optional)

Directions:

1. Soak almonds in a bowl of warm, non-chlorinated water, 18 hours, drained and rinsed. This removes the phytic acid. Drain off the water. Save the nuts for the recipe.
2. Blend soaked almonds with 3 cups of fresh, non-chlorinated water until smooth.
3. Strain mixture through a sprout bag, cheesecloth, or strainer into a big bowl.
4. The milk like liquid from the almonds is the almond milk.
5. Store in a glass container with a tight lid, in the refrigerator.

Variations:

1. For another type of sweetener, take a vanilla bean, split it, and scrape out the seeds. Add the seeds to the almond milk in the blender. Then add two or three pitted dates and blend until smooth.

2. Use a flavored stevia (Sweet Leaf brand has toffee and vanilla flavors).
3. Substitute walnuts for almonds.

Notes:

1. This milk will last in the refrigerator for about three to five days. Shake well before using.
2. Save the almond pulp in a container and put in the refrigerator or freezer for later use. I use it to make my raw breads and crackers.
3. Soaking nuts in water helps remove the phytic acid. If you want to do it even more completely, add a ¼ tsp. of organic, unpasteurized apple cider vinegar or 1 tsp. of whey to the soaking water.

Serves one to two.

◆ ◆ ◆

When experimenting with different nut milks, I found I like the creamy texture of cashews. You can make all kinds of wonderful recipes with this mixture as milk. I soak the nuts overnight in the refrigerator, but if you soak them a minimum of two hours, they will get soft enough to make a nice milk when mixed in the blender. I add extra water to make it less creamy and milkier. This mixture is great with granola cereals. I try to keep a fresh mixture of this in my refrigerator at all times. I make it fresh about every three days. By adding other flavors, it can make a nice cream for desserts and cereal toppings.

You can make any amount of this. This recipe makes a small amount (about ½ cup) to start, and you can double that easily.

CASHEW CREAM OR MILK

Ingredients:

1 c. organic cashews, preferably raw and organic

1½ c. non-chlorinated water (for soaking the nuts at least 18 hours or overnight)

½ c. non-chlorinated water (for adding to blender for cream, or 1 cup for milk)

Directions:

1. Drain nuts after soaking in 1½ c. water for18 hours or overnight. Drain nuts.
2. Blend nuts and ½ c. fresh water in blender until smooth and creamy.
3. Add water to the desired consistency. (Add the amount of liquid as you go. You can make it thicker, like a cream, or you can make it thinner, like milk.)

Note:

Soaking nuts in water helps remove the phytic acid. If you want to do it even more completely, add a ¼ tsp. of apple cider vinegar or 1 tsp. of whey to the soaking water.

Variations:

1. For a sweeter cream, add a date or two with the pit removed that has been soaked in just enough water to cover at least 30 minutes. Always add soaking water to the blender as well as dates.
2. For a sweet flavor, add Sweet Leaf brand stevia sweetener, which comes in many flavors. It has no calories and is healthy. This is my sweetener of choice. In this cream, I love the toffee flavor. Vanilla is also good.

3. Add a dash of vanilla extract, maple extract, or almond extract.
4. Use coconut water to soak the cashews and add as the water for a wonderful coconut cream.
5. Add a tablespoon or more of fruit, like some apple with a dash of cinnamon or some orange slices (with a grated zest of the rind for a bolder flavor). Ceylon cinnamon tastes good with the orange flavor; you could do lemon or lime as well. With the lemon or lime, you may want to add a tiny bit of stevia, or if the children is over 18 months, you can add a tiny bit of raw, local honey or a few more dates (which have vitamin B's).

Serves one to two.

◆ ◆ ◆

Oat milk is like rice milk only I use uncooked oats and non-flavored stevia.

OAT MILK

Ingredients:

½ c. organic, raw, gluten-free, sprouted, whole oats
1½ c. non-chlorinated water
1 vanilla bean or ¼ tsp. vanilla extract
Stevia to taste (optional)
Dash of unrefined sea salt

Directions:

1. Soak oats for 12 hours in 1 cup of the water called for in the ingredient list. This will help remove phytic acid. Pour off any water when it is finished soaking and rinse with non-chlorinated water.
2. Split vanilla bean and use a sharp knife to scrape out the inside of the bean. Put scrapings in a blender.
3. Combine all ingredients in a blender and blend well.

4. Strain through a nut milk bag or simply drink as a thicker, more fiber-filled version.

Note:

You can purchase sprouted, raw, organic oats from Blue Mountain Organics.

Variations:

1. Add more oats for a thicker milk.
2. Omit or use an alternative vanilla flavor for this milk, such as flavored stevia.
3. Add a handful or a few tablespoons of pine nuts or walnuts for a richer flavor.

Serves one to two.

◆ ◆ ◆

This is much like rice milk except with pine nuts. You can use no sweetener or no flavored stevia, if you want to use this in a recipe. This is a thin nut milk, but you can add a few more nuts to make it thicker.

Mediterranean pine nuts have more protein than any other nut. Pine nuts also have a unique ability to make you feel full and satisfied. They are great to have in the diet, especially if you need weight control. Pine nuts can be expensive, but a little goes a long way.

PINE NUT MILK

Ingredients:

1 vanilla bean

½ c. organic raw pine nuts, soaked in non-chlorinated water for 18 hours or overnight and drained

1½ c. non-chlorinated water

Stevia to taste

Dash of sea salt

Directions:

1. Split vanilla bean and use a sharp knife to scrape out the inside of the bean. Put scrapings in blender.
2. Combine all ingredients in blender and blend well.
3. Strain through a nut milk bag, or simply drink.

Variation:

Omit the vanilla bean or use an alternative vanilla flavor. (I love toffee or vanilla-flavored liquid stevia in this drink.)

Note:

1. This is a thin milk. If you want the milk thicker, use less water or use more pine nuts.
2. Soaking nuts in water helps remove the phytic acid. If you want to do it even more completely, add a ¼ tsp. of organic, unpasteurized apple cider vinegar or 1 tsp. of whey to the soaking water.

Serves one to two.

VEGAN EGG NOG

Ingredients:

1½ c. vanilla-flavored, sweet almond, hazelnut, or rice milk
1 organic banana
Pinch of nutmeg
A few drops stevia (optional)

Directions:

Place all ingredients in a blender and blend until creamy.

Note:

This recipe is easy to double. Serves one to two.

Flavors and Sweeteners for Non-Dairy Milks

For all of these milks, you can make them flavored if you wish. Here are a few ways to make them sweeter or more flavored:

- Sweet Leaf brand stevia comes in flavors including orange, vanilla, and toffee. They have no calories and are healthy. This is my sweetener of choice.
- Add a dash or more of vanilla extract, maple extract, or almond extract.
- Add a dash of Ceylon cinnamon or a little grated orange zest for a bolder flavor. Cinnamon tastes good with orange, and you can do lemon or lime as well. With lemon or lime, you may want to add a tiny bit of maple syrup, honey, or a few more dates.
- You can make many different flavors by adding any infused water.
- Coconut water can be used to soak the cashews and added to the water for a wonderful coconut cream.
- Add a bit of vanilla to this mixture.

CHAPTER 15

Recipes

The foods and recipes that follow are my favorites, especially if you want to make pureed baby food. They can be blended until smooth and creamy to suit babies or small children. Even when they're not blended, they make wonderful meals and side dishes for the whole family.

Recipes That Make Great Baby Food

Whole, organic, fresh, seasonal vegetables and fruit are the best foods for your baby. You can use my recipes as a basic guide and expand with them as you see fit. Food works in a symphonic way. The combination can be beautiful, healing and harmonious.

I add unrefined sea salt to some of these recipes; so the food has more electrolytes and minerals. The unrefined, sea salt also aids the body in absorbing minerals like potassium from the food and aids in hydrating the body, when drinking purified drinking water.

I also add some healthy fats to these recipes to support brain health and provide energy. As the child grows you can adjust the amount of healthy fats, like coconut oil for the diet. A growing teenager may need about a tablespoon or more of unrefined, organic coconut oil or cold pressed flax or hemp seed oil or an avocado, depending on his activity level.

Avocado is a perfect food. The avocado is a great source of potassium, Vitamin K, B, C, E and fiber. One avocado has around 4 grams of protein. The avocado is also a great source of monounsaturated fat, which is considered a good fat. They are a nutritious addition to any diet.

I added organic sprouts and some fresh, seasonal, organic, raw fruits or vegetables (I happen to have in my garden or kitchen) to my recipes when I was making my own baby food. This adds fresh enzymes, extra nutrients and some variety to the child's diet. I highly recommend this. If you are feeling bold, use my recipes as a guide and you can create your own fabulous dishes from them.

In this group of recipes, almost all are vegan, vegetarian, raw, and gluten-free.

Meals You Can Make for Everyone

Vegan/vegetarian/gluten-free

STEAMED BROCCOLI

Ingredients:

1 c. organic broccoli (cut into bite-sized pieces)

⅛ tsp. unrefined sea salt

¼ tsp. pure organic coconut oil

1 T. pure water

Directions:

1. Slightly steam broccoli until just bright green and soft. Steam just a minute!
2. Serve warm with the salt and coconut oil drizzled over it.
3. For baby food that is pureed, place broccoli, salt, water and coconut oil in blender or food processor and blend until creamy smooth. You can also add one-fourth of a freshly peeled and pitted organic avocado (to this food processor mixture) for the baby food. It makes it even creamier and more nutritious.

Note:

You can add more water to create the consistency you desire.

Serves one to two.

Vegan/vegetarian/raw/gluten-free

FRESH SQUASH

Ingredients:

1 c. fresh organic zucchini or crooked neck squash (grated or shredded)

⅛ tsp. unrefined sea salt

¼ tsp. pure organic extra virgin olive oil or coconut oil

Directions:

1. Place the grated squash in a bowl. Combine the oil well with the squash.
2. Serve with unrefined sea salt lightly sprinkled over it.
3. For baby food that is pureed, place the squash/zucchini, salt, water and oil in blender or food processor and blend until creamy smooth. You can also add one-fourth of a freshly peeled and pitted organic avocado (to this food processor mixture) for the baby food. It makes it even creamier and more nutritious.

Note:

You can add a little water to create the consistency you desire.

Serves one to two.

◆ ◆ ◆

Vegan/vegetarian/gluten-free

STEAMED BROCCOLI AND QUINOA

Ingredients:

1 c. organic broccoli crowns (cut into bite-sized pieces)

1 c. cooked organic quinoa

¼ tsp. unrefined sea salt

½ tsp. pure organic coconut oil

Directions:

1. Steam broccoli, for about one minute, just until bright green.
2. Place broccoli, cooked quinoa, salt and coconut oil in a pan and sauté a few minutes until the flavors meld together. Serve warm.
3. For baby food that is pureed, place the broccoli and quinoa, salt, water and coconut oil in blender or food processor and blend until creamy smooth.

Note:

You can add a little non-chlorinated water or alternative milk to create the consistency you desire.

Variations:

Substitute cooked, sprouted lentils and rice for the quinoa.

Serves two or three.

◆ ◆ ◆

Vegan/vegetarian/gluten-free

SQUASH AND STEAMED CARROTS

Ingredients:

1 organic zucchini or crooked neck squash (cut into ½ inch chunks or grated)

1 c. organic carrots with the skin on; cut into ½-inch chunks

¼ tsp. unrefined sea salt

1 tsp. organic, extra-virgin olive oil

Directions:

1. Steam carrots until just slightly soft.
2. Toss the carrots and zucchini in oil and salt until lightly coated.
3. Serve room temperature or slightly warm.

4. For baby food that is pureed, place the squash, carrots, salt and coconut oil in blender or food processor and blend until creamy smooth. You can also add one-fourth of a freshly peeled and pitted organic avocado (to this food processor mixture) for the baby food. It makes it even creamier and more nutritious.

Note:

You can add a little water to create the consistency you desire.

Serves one to two.

◆ ◆ ◆

Vegan/vegetarian/ gluten-free

STEAMED BROCCOLI AND RICE

Ingredients:

1 c. organic broccoli crowns (cut into bite-sized pieces)
1 c. cooked, organic, whole grain, brown rice
½ tsp. unrefined sea salt
½ tsp. pure organic coconut oil
½ tsp. cold-pressed organic flax or hemp seed oil

Directions:

1. Steam broccoli just a moment until just barely soft.
2. Place broccoli, cooked whole grain brown rice, salt and coconut oil in a pan and sauté a few minutes until the flavors meld together.
3. Remove from heat and stir in the flax or hemp seed oil.
4. Serve warm.
5. For baby food that is pureed, place the broccoli, cooked whole grain brown rice, salt and coconut oil and flax or hemp seed oil in blender or food processor and blend until creamy smooth.

Note:

You can add a little non-chlorinated water to create the consistency you desire.

Variation:

Substitute quinoa for rice.

Serves two to three.

◆ ◆ ◆

Vegan/vegetarian/gluten-free

GREEN BEANS AND RICE

Ingredients:

1 c. fresh organic, green beans (cut into bite-sized pieces)
1 c. cooked, organic, whole grain, brown rice
¼ tsp. unrefined sea salt
½ tsp. pure organic coconut oil
½ tsp. cold pressed, organic flax or hemp seed oil

Directions:

1. Use green beans raw or steam the green beans until barely soft.
2. Place green beans, cooked whole grain brown rice, salt and coconut oil in a pan and sauté a few minutes until the flavors meld together.
3. Remove from heat and stir in the flax or hemp seed oil.
4. Serve warm.
5. For baby food that is pureed, place the green beans, cooked whole grain brown rice, salt and coconut oil and flax or hemp seed oil in blender or food processor and blend until creamy smooth. You can also add one-fourth of a freshly peeled and pitted organic avocado (to this food processor mixture) for the baby food. It makes it even creamier and more nutritious.

Variations:

1. Substitute quinoa for rice or snow peas for the green beans.
2. Add a little ghee to it for a buttery flavor.

Note:

You can add a little water to create the consistency you desire.
Serves two to three.

◆ ◆ ◆

Vegan/vegetarian/gluten-free

SAUTÉED CARROTS

Ingredients:

1 c. organic carrots (cut into small slices)
1 T. organic coconut oil
1 tsp. organic ghee (optional)
¼ tsp. whole, unrefined sea salt

Directions:

1. Sauté carrots and coconut oil until carrots are just tender.
2. Add ghee and keep on heat until it is melted.
3. Sprinkle with sea salt and serve warm.
4. For baby food that is pureed, place in a blender or process in a food processor until creamy. You can also add one-fourth of a freshly peeled and pitted organic avocado (to this food processor mixture) for the baby food. It makes it even creamier and more nutritious.

Note:

You can add a little water to create the consistency you desire.
Serves one to two.

Vegan/vegetarian/gluten-free

STEAMED CARROTS

Ingredients:

1 c. organic carrots (cut into bite-sized slices)
¼ tsp. whole, unrefined sea salt
½ tsp. organic coconut oil

Directions:

1. Steam carrots until carrots are just tender.
2. Sprinkle with sea salt and drizzle with the coconut oil.
3. Serve warm.
4. For baby food that is pureed, place the carrots, sea salt and coconut oil in a food processor and blend until creamy smooth. You can also add one-fourth of a freshly peeled and pitted organic avocado (to this food processor mixture) for the baby food. It makes it even creamier and more nutritious.

Serves one to two.

◆ ◆ ◆

Vegan/vegetarian/raw/gluten-free

WATERMELON

Watermelon is packed with electrolytes and is extremely hydrating. Adding sea salt helps your body absorb more of the potassium in the watermelon.

You can serve any kind of fresh, seasonal fruit like this to your child. Fresh, seasonal fruit is a delicious, hydrating way to nourish your child.

Ingredients:

2 c. organic watermelon
¼ tsp. unrefined, whole sea salt

Directions:

1. Cut watermelon into bite sized pieces.
2. Sprinkle lightly with whole, sea salt.
3. For babies, you will blend this up in a blender and serve in a bottle. For larger children, let them try eating this. It almost melts in your mouth.

Note:

This makes a good food when someone is dehydrated or constipated. Serves one to two.

Breakfast Foods

Simple, real, nutrient-dense foods served with love.

Vegan/vegetarian/gluten-free

OATMEAL WITH RAISINS

This oatmeal with raisins recipe makes a good baby food when blended or pureed, but when it's not blended, it's a great breakfast for anyone. This needs to be started the day before you want to serve it. This recipe doubles easily.

Ingredients:

1 c. pure water
½ c. dry, gluten-free, organic, sprouted, whole oats
Pinch of ground Ceylon ground cinnamon
¼ tsp. unrefined sea salt
½ tsp. cold pressed organic hemp seed oil
½ tsp. pure unrefined coconut oil
¼ c. raisins

Directions:

1. Soak oats overnight in non-chlorinated warm water and rinse.
2. Soak raisins in water until plump.
3. Put water in a saucepan and bring to a boil.
4. Add the oats, salt and coconut oil and bring to a boil.
5. Cook 4 to 5 minutes, stirring frequently.
6. Remove from heat.
7. Add raisins and cinnamon and stir.
8. Add the hemp oil and stir.
9. Serve warm

Variation:

1. You can add ½ tsp. of xylitol for a sweeter version.
2. For extra nutrition, add a teaspoon of raw, sprouted apricot seed butter to the dish before serving.

Note:

1. If serving this to a baby or small child, mix it in a food processor or blender until smooth and creamy. You may need to add a little milk or water if it's too thick.
2. You can purchase sprouted, raw, organic, gluten-free oats and sprouted seed butter from Blue Mountain Organics.

Serves one to two.

◆ ◆ ◆

Vegetarian/gluten-free

SCRAMBLED EGGS

When my children were growing up, I'd give them a good breakfast before they left for school. Eggs have been found to make people feel fuller and more satisfied longer, maybe because of the protein content. I would give my children smoothies with high protein content and scrambled eggs or oatmeal and they would be able to last at school until lunch.

Buy organic, humanely raised, fresh eggs from chickens that are kept in open, fresh-air, sunny, green-grass pasture environments. You may want to find a local farmer you can trust from whom you can buy your eggs.

Ingredients:

2–3 organic, humanely and pasture raised eggs
2 T. milk of choice
1 or 2 T. organic coconut oil
Unrefined, sea salt to taste

Directions:

1. Beat eggs in a bowl with milk.
2. Heat oil in a skillet over medium heat.
3. Put eggs in the skillet and stir until eggs are cooked to your liking.
4. Add salt and pepper to taste.
5. For babies, place in a blender and blend until it is smooth enough to serve a baby.

Variations:

1. Add baby spinach, chopped tomatoes, and/or mushrooms.
2. Make this as an omelet: Don't stir eggs when they are in the pan. Let cook, and then gently fold over and slide out of the pan onto a plate.

Note:

Use a little more oil (a teaspoon or more) if you are cooking more than four eggs.

Serves one to two.

◆ ◆ ◆

Vegetarian/gluten-free

SCRAMBLED EGGS WITH BABY SPINACH

The ingredients listed for scrambled eggs with spinach are for two small children or one adult serving. I use baby spinach.

Ingredients:

2–3 organic, humanely and pasture raised eggs

2 T. organic milk of choice (coconut milk works well)

1 or 2 T. organic coconut oil

1 small organic scallion (finely chopped)

½ c. of organic baby spinach

Unrefined, pure sea salt to taste

Directions:

1. Beat eggs in a bowl with milk.
2. Heat 1 T. Oil in a skillet over medium heat.
3. Sauté the scallion and the baby spinach a minute and then remove and set aside for a minute.
4. Put 1 T. more of coconut oil in the skillet and add the eggs to the skillet and stir until eggs are almost cooked to your liking.
5. Add the baby spinach and scallion and stir another minute.
6. Add unrefined sea salt to taste.
7. For a baby food or a small child, place about a cup of this finished food in the food processor with a few tablespoons of alternative milk such as coconut milk and blend until creamy.
8. Serve warm.

Variations:

1. Add chopped tomatoes.
2. To make this as an omelet, don't stir eggs when they are in the pan. Let it cook, and add the baby spinach when it is almost done and then gently fold over and slide out of the pan onto a plate.

Note:

Buy organic, humanely raised, fresh eggs from chickens kept in open, fresh-air, sunny, green-grass pasture environments.

Serves one to two.

Vegan/vegetarian/gluten-free

APPLE QUINOA

You must start this recipe the day before you want to serve it.

Ingredients:

2 c. pure water

1 c. organic, whole-grain, sprouted quinoa

1 tsp. pure vanilla extract

¼ c. organic unsweetened almond or coconut milk

1 apple, cored, and grated

1 tsp. xylitol or a few drops of stevia to sweeten (optional)

1 tsp. Ceylon cinnamon

¼ tsp. Unrefined sea salt

Directions:

1. Soak the quinoa 18 hours or overnight in non-chlorinated water (then drain).
2. Put the quinoa and 1 cup water and sea salt into a medium cooking pan and bring to a boil.
3. Cover, reduce heat to medium low and simmer until water is absorbed, 15 to 20 minutes.
4. Add vanilla.
5. Add almond milk and stir.
6. Remove from heat.
7. Combine the xylitol and the cinnamon (if using).
8. Mix in grated apple and xylitol (if using) and cinnamon.
9. Serve warm.

Serves one to two (about ½ cup each).

Note:

1. Soaking seeds (like quinoa) in water helps remove the phytic acid. If you want to do it even more completely, add a ¼ tsp. of apple cider vinegar or 1 tsp. of whey to the soaking water.

2. You can purchase sprouted quinoa from Blue Mountain Organics.

◆ ◆ ◆

Vegan/vegetarian/raw/gluten-free

CHIA SEED PUDDING WITH NUT CRÈME TOPPING

Start this chia seed pudding recipe the day before you wish to serve it. This recipe is for two or more servings; it can easily be doubled. This makes a delicious and healthy desert as well.

Ingredients:

1 c. organic chia seeds
3½ c. purified water
¼ dropper of liquid stevia
Fresh organic blueberries (or berries of choice) and/or sliced bananas (to add to the pudding; optional)

Directions for the pudding:

1. Soak chia seeds in 3½ c. water in a very large bowl (these seeds expand greatly) overnight in the refrigerator. Make sure you cover them with at least 3 inches of water. The chia seeds get soft and expand, which makes the pudding. Add more water as necessary. Stir if you get a chance.
2. The next day, take pudding out of refrigerator and gently mix in the stevia and then add in berries or banana slices. Combine gently.
3. Place chia pudding in individual serving bowls.
4. Serve this with the nut crème topping

Note:

If serving this to a baby or small child, mix it in a food processor or blender until smooth and creamy. If it's too thick, you may need to add a little alternative milk or water.

NUT CRÈME TOPPING

Ingredients:

½ to ¾ cup organic pine nuts or cashews

2 c. purified water or coconut water

A few drops stevia (plain, toffee-flavored, or vanilla-flavored)

Directions for the cashew or pine nut crème:

1. Soak cashews or pine nuts in 1 c. non-chlorinated water for 18 hours or overnight. Pour off soaking water. The soaking water contains the phytic acid that we wanted to remove. The nuts are much more digestible when the phytic acid is removed.
2. Add 1 c. of clean, new water to blender (you can use coconut water).
3. Blend cashews or pine nuts and water with stevia, adding more water if you want it thinner. (I prefer it thick like a crème.) Make sure it is extremely creamy smooth. Top each bowl of pudding with a dollop of cashew or pine nut crème.

Notes:

1. For a baby food or a small child, place about a cup of this finished food in the blender with a few tablespoons of alternative milk (e.g., coconut milk) and blend until extremely creamy and smooth.
2. SweetLeaf brand stevia comes in flavors like vanilla, orange, and toffee. They are good for flavoring nut milks and crèmes. I usually find them at the healthy grocery store in the baking section or in the sweetener section.

Serves two to three.

Vegetarian/gluten-free

AMANDA'S BACK FROM AFRICA WAFFLES

I grew up eating waffles, so I frequently made them for my children. The week my daughter came home from the Peace Corps in Africa, we decided to make waffles. I had this wonderful freshly ground organic buckwheat flour from the farmers' market so we used it. My daughter said that in Africa, she made pancakes from the mix I sent her. Since they didn't have any maple syrup, she used honey.

We ate our waffles with honey and cinnamon that morning. Amanda also wanted to add some dried cranberries to the batter. They tasted delicious in our waffles. The cranberries are optional. We added about a ¼ cup of them to our batter.

Ingredients for about three 9-inch waffles:

2 cups organic, whole grain, sprouted buckwheat flour (sifted)
2 T. xylitol (a natural sugar I use when the recipe calls for granulated sugar)
3 tsp. baking powder (aluminum-free)
¾ tsp. sea salt
1½ cups organic coconut milk
3 organic, humane, pasture raised eggs (separated)
¼ c. coconut oil (melted)
¼ c. dried, organic cranberries (optional)
Dash Ceylon cinnamon (optional)
Drizzle of maple syrup or honey (no honey for anyone under 18 months) (optional)
A few tablespoons of melted butter (optional)

Directions:

1. Heat up the waffle iron.
2. Sift the flour, sugar, baking powder and salt into a bowl.
3. Combine milk and egg yolks and beat in the coconut oil.

4. Add the liquid ingredients to the dry ingredients and stir lightly.
5. Beat the egg whites until they will form soft peaks.
6. Fold the egg whites into the batter.
7. Bake the waffles for about 5 minutes (time may vary with various waffle irons).
8. Serve with melted butter (optional), honey or maple syrup with a dash of cinnamon (optional) sprinkled on top.

Variations:

1. Add about ¼ cup of blueberries or banana pieces instead of the cranberries, to the batter for a fruitier version.
2. Use flour such as spelt or another gluten-free flour such as coconut, quinoa or oat flour.
3. For a vegan version, you can use 1 T. freshly ground flax or chia (chia seeds don't have to be ground) seeds mixed with 3 T. of water for each egg. Then refrigerate the flax/water mixture for 15 minutes before adding to the waffle mixture. Just add it to the mixture where it calls for egg yolks. You won't be able to do this recipe exactly, but it does work nicely.

Note:

You can purchase sprouted flours, like buckwheat, from Blue Mountain Organics. See resources. Sprouted flours have less (if any) phytic acid in them.

Makes about three waffles.

Vegetarian/gluten-free

RASPBERRY MUFFINS

I was talking to my children about my book and they both said, "Mom, you're putting in the raspberry muffins, aren't you?" This is one of their absolute favorite breakfasts. Making them is easy, and they are delicious. I'd frequently double or even triple this recipe because they always wanted more!

Ingredients:

1 c. organic, sprouted quinoa or teff flour
1 c. organic, non-GMO whole, yellow corn flour
1 c. fresh organic raspberries
2 T. melted organic ghee or butter (melted)
3 T. organic, pure coconut oil (melted)
½ cup organic plain yogurt (coconut will work fine)
½ tsp. unrefined sea salt
½ c. fine grain xylitol
1 tsp. baking powder
½ tsp. baking soda
1 organic egg
½ cup organic, orange juice
¼ tsp. organic, grated orange rind

Directions:

1. Preheat oven at 400 degrees F.
2. Use one of the tablespoons of coconut oil to grease the 12 large muffin cups with it.
3. In a mixing bowl, combine all the dry (flours, baking soda, baking powder, salt, and xylitol) ingredients well.
4. In another mixing bowl, combine all the egg, melted butter or ghee, melted coconut oil, yogurt, orange juice, and orange rind and mix well.

5. Gently pour the wet ingredient combination into the middle of the dry ingredients, but making a kind of well in the center. Then blend quickly.
6. Gently add the raspberries and fold them in quickly. Don't over mix.
7. Pour the batter quickly and gently into the muffin cups. Fill them about half full.
8. Bake for 15 to 20 minutes. Depending on the altitude and the size of your muffin cups. The muffins should be a toasty color when ready.

Notes:

1. You can use frozen berries, they don't taste quite as good, but make sure to defrost them and drain off any juice before adding them.
2. You can purchase sprouted flours, like buckwheat, from Blue Mountain Organics. See resources. Sprouted flours have less (if any) phytic acid in them.

Makes 6 to 12 muffins.

Soups

Soups are easy to make especially in large batches. I would frequently make a double recipe, if I had a large enough pot. I save some in the refrigerator for the next day or freeze it and use it as a meal another day.

All of these soup recipes are vegan, vegetarian, and gluten-free. They are easily turned into a baby food consistency when placed in a blender. For older children or adults, I would serve them with some whole grain breads and it would be a whole meal.

Vegetarian/gluten-free

ASPARAGUS-POTATO SOUP

This soup is one of my children's absolute favorite soups. A woman from India shared this recipe with me as we watched our daughters practice gymnastics. I changed it a little bit over the years. Everyone who eats it loves it.

Milk makes the soup richer and creamier. Some of the milks I use in my recipe is vanilla coconut milk or almond milk. I leave the skins on the potatoes in this recipe.

Ingredients:

1 organic onion, chopped in large pieces
2 T. organic ghee, butter, or extra-virgin, pure coconut oil
1 bunch organic asparagus
3 large organic sweet potatoes
6 c. water
1 tsp. sea salt
1 c. unsweetened organic milk (any variety)

Directions:

1. Sauté onion in ghee, butter, or oil in a large soup pot, until onion starts to look a little clear.

2. Cut off and discard hard ends of the asparagus (about a half inch).
3. Cut asparagus and potatoes in large chunks.
4. Add asparagus to onion mixture and sauté a moment more.
5. Add water, potatoes, and sea salt, and bring to a boil.
6. Reduce heat and cook over medium heat until potatoes are tender.
7. Remove from heat.
8. When soup is cooler, blend mixture in blender until creamy and smooth.
9. Add milk, if using.

Variation:

Use another type of potato. The original recipe called for russet potatoes, but any variety is delicious. I love the sweet potato flavor, and sweet potatoes have color. Purple potatoes taste great, but they look a little purple!

Notes:

1. For a baby food or a smaller child, place about a cup in the blender and blend until creamy.
2. Be careful when blending hot ingredients. The steam and heat can build up, and it can explode though the top of the blender, burning you and making a terrible mess. I always do it carefully with small amounts. I also cover the blender with a large dish towel to help protect me (and the kitchen) from a mess.

Serves six to eight.

Vegan/vegetarian/gluten-free

SPLIT PEA SOUP

Ingredients:

2 c. organic split peas

8 c. cold water

2 organic stalks celery, chopped

2 medium organic carrots, chopped

2 small organic onions, chopped

1 tsp. whole, unrefined sea salt

1 Tbsp. fresh organic parsley sprigs to use as garnish when serving (optional)

1 T. organic coconut oil

Directions:

1. Rinse the split peas several times and make sure there aren't little stones in there. Set aside a minute.
2. Place coconut oil, chopped onion, carrot, and celery in a large pot and sauté about 8 minutes.
3. Add the peas and water to the pot and bring to a boil over medium heat. Then let it simmer for about 35 minutes or until the split peas are soft.
4. You can eat it as a chunky soup or put it in a blender and blend it until creamy.

Notes:

1. For a baby food, place about a cup of this in the blender or food processor and blend until creamy.
2. This makes a large pot of soup that can serve about 8 people. This soup can be refrigerated for future meals.

Serves four to six.

Vegan/vegetarian/gluten-free

BLACK BEAN SOUP

This black bean soup recipe is an easy one that you can cook in a slow cooker. If you want a warm meal when you get home from being out all day, this rich and satisfying dish is a great choice. Serve it with whole grain bread for a wonderful family supper.

Ingredients:

1½ c. organic black beans (soaked 18 hours in non-chlorinated water and drained)

10–12 c. water

1 organic red onion, diced

3 stalks celery, chopped into half-inch chunks

3 organic carrots, chopped into bite sized chunks

2 T. organic, extra-virgin pure coconut oil

2 vegetable bouillon cubes

1 c. hot water

2 small organic, garlic cloves, minced

1 tsp. sea salt

1 tsp. organic parsley

½ tsp. organic oregano

½ tsp. organic thyme

Directions:

1. Soak beans overnight in water.
2. Pour off water.
3. Sauté onion, celery, and carrots 5 minutes in oil. Place in slow cooker.
4. Bring beans and about 4 cups of water (enough water to cover them) to a boil, and then drain off water.
5. In a small dish, dissolve bouillon cubes in 1-cup hot water.

6. Place beans in slow cooker with remaining ingredients, including dissolved bouillon, 6 additional cups of water, and herbs and spices.
7. Turn on slow cooker and cook 6–8 hours on low.

Variations:

1. When soaking beans, make sure you put them in a very large dish and the water covers beans by at least 2 or 3 inches. Beans will double or triple in size as they soak overnight. When they are finished soaking, drain off the water and use fresh water for cooking. I change out the cooking water twice. I do this because it removes the phytic acid and makes the beans more digestible.
2. Serve with a big dollop of thick, plain organic yogurt, or sour cream.
3. Sprinkle with chopped parsley and chives as garnish.

Notes:

1. For a baby food or a smaller child, place about a cup of the finished soup in the blender and blend until creamy.
2. Soaking beans in water helps remove the phytic acid. If you want to do it even more completely, add a ¼ tsp. of apple cider vinegar or 1 tsp. of whey to the soaking water.

Serves four to six.

◆ ◆ ◆

Vegetarian/gluten-free

LENTIL SOUP

My children adore this soup and are always asking me to make it when they are home. I start this soup the day before I want to serve it, so I have time to soak my lentils. This helps remove the phytic acid.

Serve this with crusty whole-grain bread.

Ingredients:

1 c. organic sprouted lentils (if you don't have sprouted lentils, then soak the lentils for 18 hours in non-chlorinated water and then drain)
2 T. organic extra-virgin, pure coconut oil
2 organic onions, chopped
3 organic carrots, chopped
¾ tsp. organic marjoram
¾ tsp. organic thyme
½ tsp. salt (or to taste)
¼ tsp. black pepper
3 c. organic tomatoes (crushed or diced)
7 c. pure, non chlorinated water
⅓ c. fresh or 2 T. dried organic parsley
½ c. or more grated organic cheddar cheese (optional–leave out for vegan choice or use a vegan cheese)

Directions:

1. Sauté oil, onions, carrots, marjoram, thyme, salt, and pepper about 4–5 minutes in a large soup pot.
2. Add tomatoes and stir for a couple of minutes.
3. Add water and lentils.
4. Bring to a boil, then reduce heat to a simmer and cook 45 minutes, or until lentils are soft.
5. Remove from heat and add parsley.
6. Sprinkle with cheese, if using.

Notes:

1. For a baby food, place about a cup of the finished soup in the blender and blend until creamy.
2. Soaking lentils and/or beans in water helps remove the phytic acid. If you want to do it even more completely,

add a ¼ tsp. of apple cider vinegar or 1 tsp. of whey to the soaking water.

Serves four to six.

◆ ◆ ◆

Vegan/vegetarian/raw/gluten-free

RAW TOMATO BASIL SOUP

Ingredients:

2 cups organic tomatoes, chopped

2 sun-dried tomatoes (soaked in olive oil or water to soften)

½ small organic garlic clove, minced

2 fresh leaves of organic basil or a ¼ tsp. dried

1 half of an organic cucumber, chopped

½ small organic scallion, chopped (about ¼ tsp.)

½ tsp. organic coconut oil

½ avocado (peeled and pitted)

½ tsp. whole sea salt (to taste)

Directions:

Blend all ingredients in blender until well blended.

Serves two.

◆ ◆ ◆

Vegan/vegetarian/raw/gluten-free

CUCUMBER SOUP

This is a nutrient packed soup that is refreshing. I like to serve it on hot summer days.

It makes a great snack and is good to serve to small children as a meal. This is an easy dish to prepare for maximum health benefits. This is a easy way to get super healthy green food into a child's diet, especially if they can't chew food yet. This recipe makes about 2 servings. I estimate one cup per person. This recipe is easily doubled or tripled.

Ingredients:

1 cucumber, peeled and chopped into chunks
1 avocado, peeled and pitted
1 cup romaine lettuce, chopped
Juice of half a lemon (freshly squeezed)
¼ tsp of freshly grated lemon rind
½ cup pure, non-chlorinated water
1/2 tsp. unrefined sea salt
1 tsp. fresh dill (fresh is best, but dried will work fine) or ½ tsp. dried dill (taste it, you may like more dill in yours)

Directions:

Place all ingredients in the blender and blend until smooth. Note: If it seems to thick, add a little more water.

Variation:

1. Use cilantro as the herb instead of the dill.

Note:

This soup should keep about 2 days in the refrigerator.

◆ ◆ ◆

This is an easy, delicious, high-protein, nutrient rich, and probiotic-rich soup. I frequently make this to sip in the afternoon instead of afternoon tea.

Vegan/vegetarian/gluten-free

MISO SOUP WITH MUSHROOMS

Ingredients:

10 dried organic shitake mushrooms, sliced
4½ c. non-chlorinated water
¼ c. organic miso
¼ c. chopped organic watercress for garnish (optional)

Directions:

1. Soak mushrooms at least 10 minutes in ½ cup water, until soft.
2. Simmer 4 cups water in a pan. Do not boil.
3. Add miso and stir until miso is dissolved.
4. Remove from heat.
5. Add mushrooms and their soaking liquid when miso water is just warm enough to drink.

Variation:

1. Add kombu seaweed for additional nutrition.
2. You can use whatever mushrooms you prefer.

Note:

For a baby food, place about a cup of the finished soup in the blender and blend until creamy. You can add a little fresh avocado to this to make it creamier.

Serves two to four.

◆ ◆ ◆

Vegan/vegetarian/gluten-free

NUTRITIOUS BROTH WITH MUSHROOMS AND GARLIC

Sunny, an acupuncturist I know, once told me to make a soup using zucchini, carrots, celery, potatoes (I like to use colored ones such as purple or sweet) and a sweet onion. I started making this broth and then added seaweed as well. I drain off the vegetables after I make it and drink the broth.

You can save the vegetables and eat them, or eat it all together as a vegetable soup. I add the garlic last because it is fragile. Garlic has anticancer properties; it may decrease the risk of breast, colon, stomach, throat, and skin cancer. It also contains both antibiotic and antifungal properties.

The secret to garlic's health benefits is sulfides. The sulfides aren't released unless the garlic is crushed or chopped, and then left to sit at least 10 to 15 minutes before eating. Add more garlic if you want a more medicinal soup. Drink this while it is warm.

This recipe is highly alkalizing as well.

Ingredients:

4 organic carrots cut in small chunks
½ c. organic peas
4 cups of organic green beans
1 organic zucchini cut in small chunks
2 organic celery stalks cut in small chunks
1–2 organic sweet potatoes cut in small chunks
½ organic onion cut in small chunks
2-inch-piece kombu seaweed
1 tsp. unrefined sea salt (Nancy's sensational sea salt is a good choice.)
5 c. non-chlorinated water (estimate how much you need as you fill the pot; you may need more)
1 or 2 organic cloves garlic, finely minced
¼ c. organic mushrooms, sliced (optional)

Directions:

1. Place carrots, peas, zucchini, celery, potatoes, onion, seaweed, and sea salt in a large pot with water in it and bring to a boil.
2. Reduce heat and simmer about 20 minutes, until potatoes are tender.
3. Add garlic and mushrooms and simmer 4 more minutes.
4. Strain vegetables out.
5. Serve as a broth/soup, warm.

Note:

1. For a baby food, place about a cup of the finished soup in the blender and blend until creamy.

2. You can eat this as a vegetable soup (instead of broth) or eat the vegetables as a side dish as well.

Serves two to four.

Main Dishes

The recipes in this section are for older children who chew well, responsibly, and with the use of all of their teeth. Make sure to always serve your child food that is appropriate for their teeth and swallowing ability. Almost any food can be put in a food processor and blended until smooth and creamy enough to feed a baby. Use your best judgment as to what your own child can consume. I frequently made our meals into baby food using our food processor.

You can also make many any of these recipes with vegan cheese or alternative milks, if you want to make them as a vegan version.

Vegan/vegetarian/gluten-free

POTATO, BROCCOLI, AND BEAN STEW

I love broccoli and potatoes together. Add beans, and you have a rich and hearty dish. This is actually quite easy; you can use canned beans if you need to. I like to use white northern beans, but kidney beans will work as well.

This is a nice meal to serve when entertaining because you can make it ahead of time and warm it up when you're ready to serve. Inexpensive, satisfying, easy, and full of nutrition—this stew is hard to beat.

Ingredients:

1½ lb. organic potatoes cut into 2-inch cubes (use sweet potatoes)

1 T. extra-virgin, pure coconut oil

½ tsp. unrefined, sea salt

10 c. non-chlorinated water

2 c. organic northern white beans (cooked)

2 c. organic broccoli cut in ½ to 1 inch pieces

2 Small organic garlic cloves, minced

Directions:

1. Cook potatoes, coconut oil, and sea salt in the water until potatoes are just tender. (This can take anywhere from 25 to 40 minutes.)

2. Add beans, broccoli, and garlic. Stir for a few minutes, and then simmer about 10 minutes, stirring occasionally (so that nothing burns).
3. Serve warm.

Notes:

1. For a baby food or a small child, place about a cup of this finished food in the blender with a few tablespoons of alternative milk such as unsweetened coconut milk and blend until creamy.
2. Yukon gold, purple, and sweet potatoes are all good choices.
3. This recipe can be made in a crock-pot.

Serves four to six.

◆ ◆ ◆

Vegan/vegetarian/gluten-free

WHOLE GRAIN RICE AND LENTILS

I would start this recipe the day before I want to serve it. This way, I have time to soak the rice and lentils.

Ingredients:

1 c. organic whole grain rice (sprouted)
½ c. organic lentils (sprouted)
1 T. organic coconut oil
2 ¾ c. pure, non-chlorinated water
½ tsp. unrefined sea salt

Directions:

1. Wash rice and lentils in cold water until water runs clear. (Before you mix the lentils with the rice, look at the lentils and make sure there aren't any little stones in the mix.) Note: I frequently soak my rice and lentils if they are not sprouted. I would soak them for 18 hours or overnight in non-chlorinated water and drained, to remove the phytic acid and to sprout them. This makes them

easier to digest after cooking. I drain off the water and then use new water for cooking. When I need a little less water in which to cook them in, because they are softer. So, if you soak your lentils and rice overnight (which I recommend), pour off the water you soak them in and then use about 2 cups of fresh water for cooking.

2. Place the coconut oil, sea salt, rice, and lentils in a large saucepan.
3. Add water (2 cups) to pan. It should cover the lentils and rice by about ½ inch.
4. Bring to a boil over high heat.
5. Reduce heat to medium and cover with a (see-through) lid. Allow liquid to be absorbed (about 20 - 40 minutes). When only a few bubbles remain on the surface, reduce heat to a minimum, cover tightly, and steam about 10–15 minutes without stirring. (Taste test a lentil to see if it's tender. When tender, the dish is ready)
6. Remove from heat and serve warm.

Note:

1. For a baby food, simply place the cooked rice and lentils and a little bit of water in a blender and blend until creamy.
2. For the baby food, you can add some fresh mango fruit to the blending combination.

Variation:

Add some cut up mango to this finished dish.

Serves three to four.

Vegan/ vegetarian/gluten-free

BASIC COOKED BEANS

Beans are high in fiber, protein, and flavor, plus they're inexpensive and easy to store. Be sure to store uncooked, raw beans in a dark, cool, dry place. Beans are easy to freeze and thaw, so make a large batch and freeze some to use later. Beans are easy to add to salads or serve as a side dish with soup or bread. One pound of dried beans will yield 5–6 cups of cooked beans.

The optional seaweed in this recipe adds nutrients and helps make beans more digestible.

Ingredients:

1 lb. organic dried beans (any variety)

10 c. water, plus more for soaking and cooking

2-inch piece seaweed (optional)

1 Tsp. organic, pure coconut oil

Whole unrefined sea salt to taste

Directions:

1. Check beans, and discard any that are shriveled or discolored. Also check to make sure no little stones or foreign matter are mixed in with beans.
2. Soak beans in warm, non-chlorinated water 18 hours. Make sure the dish is large enough for beans to double in size and enough water to cover them by at least 2 inches.
3. Pour off water.
4. In a 5-quart saucepan, bring 10 cups fresh, pure water and beans to a boil.
5. Discard water and keep beans.
6. Refill pot with new, purified water to about 2 inches over the top of beans. Add salt and seaweed, if using.
7. Bring water with beans to a boil again.
8. Reduce heat to a simmer, add the coconut oil and cook beans until tender (about 45 minutes to an hour, depending on the size

of beans; larger beans will take longer). Add more water if it gets too low and tops of beans are showing.

9. Remove from heat and they are ready to eat!

Notes:

1. For a baby food or a smaller child, place about a cup of the cooked beans in the blender or food processor with about 3 T. unsweetened nut milk and blend until creamy.
2. The extra-virgin, pure coconut oil adds extra richness and supports brain health, gives the body energy and helps the body know how to use the protein and carbohydrates.
3. Soaking beans/lentils in water helps remove the phytic acid. If you want to do it even more completely, add a ¼ tsp. of apple cider vinegar or 1 tsp. of whey to the soaking water.
4. You can purchase sprouted beans. If you have sprouted beans you won't need to soak the beans.

Serves three to four.

◆ ◆ ◆

Vegan/vegetarian/gluten-free

QUINOA WITH BROCCOLI

Quinoa, a nice alternative to rice, is gluten-free and a complete seed protein. The darker variety has more antioxidants in it than the lighter because the antioxidants are the color. I suggest sautéing or steaming broccoli instead of boiling it.

Start this recipe the day before you want to serve it. This allows time to soak the quinoa and remove some of the phytic acid.

Ingredients:

2 c. organic quinoa

1 organic scallion, finely chopped

4 c. pure water

½ c. organic broccoli crowns lightly steamed and then cut into bite-size pieces
2 T. organic coconut oil
Pinch of unrefined, whole sea salt to taste

Directions:

1. Soak quinoa 18 hours in non-chlorinated water and drain.
2. Rinse the quinoa well. Then cook quinoa and all of the white part of the chopped scallion in water in a pot over a medium heat 15 to 20 minutes until quinoa is soft. Remove from heat.
3. Add broccoli, remaining scallion, coconut oil, and sea salt, and toss gently for a few moments until all is warm.
4. Serve warm.

Variation:

Substitute organic ghee for the pure organic coconut oil.

Note:

1. For a baby food or a smaller child with little chewing ability, place about a cup of the finished food in the blender or food processor with about 3-4 T. unsweetened nut milk and blend until creamy.
2. Soaking beans/lentils in water helps remove the phytic acid. If you want to do it even more completely, add a ¼ tsp. of organic apple cider vinegar or 1 tsp. of whey to the soaking water.

Serves three to four.

Vegetarian/gluten-free

STUFFED TOMATOES

I love this dish. Each tomato will serve one person. Adjust the recipe accordingly for the number of people you are serving. The tomatoes are easy to save as leftovers. Simply refrigerate them and warm them up later.

Ingredients:

8 medium organic, vine-ripened tomatoes, halved lengthwise
¼ tsp. sea salt
1 c. organic parsley (fresh)
½ c. organic oregano (fresh)
1½ c. organic Parmesan cheese, finely grated
½ c. organic, whole-grain, gluten-free breadcrumbs
2 organic garlic cloves
1 organic shallot
T. extra-virgin, pure, organic coconut oil

Directions:

1. Preheat oven to 400 degrees F.
2. Core tomatoes and scoop out seeds. Reserve tomato insides.
3. Sprinkle ⅛ tsp. of the salt over the inside of tomatoes. Set aside.
4. In a food processor, combine parsley, oregano, Parmesan, bread crumbs, garlic, shallot, coconut oil, and remaining sea salt. Pulse until herbs are chopped.
5. Chop the core of the tomato you removed, minus seeds and stems, and mix into herb mixture.
6. Pack filling into tomatoes, stuffing them to the top.
7. Place tomatoes, filling side up, on a baking dish and bake until shriveled and cheese is melted, about 12–15 minutes. Remove from heat and let stand at least 5 minutes before serving.

Variation:

For more protein, add 1 cup cooked quinoa to filling before baking.

Note:

For a small child, place about a cup of this finished food in the food processor with a few tablespoons of alternative milk, like unsweetened coconut milk or structured water and process until creamy. It will be a lot like a tomato soup puree.

Serves one person per tomato; adjust accordingly.

◆ ◆ ◆

Vegan/vegetarian/gluten-free

SWEET RICE WITH LENTILS

Coconut oil, ghee, sea salt, and a vegetable bouillon cube add richness and flavor to this basic rice/lentil dish.

Start this recipe the day before you want to serve it. This allows time to soak the rice and lentils and remove some of the phytic acid.

Ingredients:

2 c. organic whole-grain medium brown rice (sprouted is best)
¼ c. organic lentils (sprouted is best)
¼ tsp. sea salt
4 c. water
1–2 vegetable bouillon cubes, dissolved in the water
1 T. extra-virgin, pure coconut oil
½ c. organic raisins
1 T. organic ghee (optional)
¼ c. organic raw coconut flakes

Directions:

1. If the rice and lentils are not sprouted, then soak the rice and lentils 18 hours in non-chlorinated water and drain. Then put them in a small-weave sieve and rinse, until they run clean.

2. Put rice, lentils, sea salt, water (with the bouillon cube dissolved in it), coconut oil, and raisins in a large pot. It should cover the rice/lentil mixture by about ½ inch.
3. Bring to a boil; reduce heat to a simmer.
4. Cover the pot and do not disturb for 25-35 minutes. (requires a longer cooking time, if the rice and lentils have not been soaked) Do not stir.
5. When it looks as if all the water is absorbed, the rice and lentils are ready.
6. Add ghee, if you choose, to rice and lentil mixture and gently toss together.
7. Gently scoop out rice and lentils and add coconut flakes.

Variation:

Add a little sautéed onion after cooking for a richer flavor.

Notes:

1. Consider soaking the rice and lentils overnight to sprout them, which makes them easier to digest after cooking. I drain off the water and then use new water for cooking. Then I need a little less water to cook them in because they are softer due to soaking them. If you soak your lentils and rice overnight (which I recommend), pour off the water you soak them in and then use about 2 cups of fresh water for cooking. As you cook it, make sure there is about ½ inch of water over the rice/lentil mixture when you start to cook it.
2. For a baby food or a smaller child, place about a cup of this in the blender with unsweetened milk or water and blend until creamy.

Serves four to six.

Vegan/vegetarian/gluten-free

NORI ROLLS WITH RICE

These easy, healthy, and delicious rolls feed your body on a deep cellular level. Seaweed adds iodine to the diet in a whole-food form. Nori kelp, which comes in sheets, can be purchased in the Asian food section of the grocery store.

Children love making food and they can have fun with this recipe. You can cut it for them or they can eat it like a long, rolled up seaweed type of tortilla roll.

The ingredients listed here make one roll.

Ingredients:

nori sheet
umeboshi paste
organic, sprouted sesame seeds (freshly ground)
whole-grain, sprouted, organic rice, cooked
1 organic avocado, cut into ½-inch thick slices
sea salt
organic carrots, julienned
organic cucumber, julienned
organic sunflower or broccoli sprouts
organic cilantro, chopped
Nama Shoyu (unpasteurized, raw, organic soy sauce)
wasabi (optional)
pickled ginger (optional)

Directions:

1. Lay out nori sheet (shiny side down) on a flat surface or a bamboo (sushi) mat.
2. Spread a thin layer of umeboshi paste on a middle section of the nori sheet all the way across, about an inch high, leaving about a half-inch border from the outside edge.
3. Sprinkle (freshly ground up) sesame seeds across the paste.

4. Spread rice in a thin layer over sesame seeds and paste, using your fingers. (Wet your fingers to make this easier.)
5. Spread avocado over rice, staying inside the edge about one-half inch.
6. Sprinkle avocado with a little sea salt.
7. Lay carrots and cucumbers in small amounts over avocado.
8. Sprinkle with sprouts and cilantro.
9. Take the end of the nori sheet right in front of you and start rolling it away from you.
10. Seal the edge with a little water.
11. Slice, using a sharp knife, into 1-inch-thick rolls.
12. Serve with organic soy sauce for dipping, if using.

Variations:

1. Mix a tiny bit of xylitol with the soy sauce to make it sweeter.
2. You may have some wasabi (optional) and /or pickled ginger (optional), if the child is older. Use your best judgment.

◆ ◆ ◆

Vegetarian/gluten-free (if the bread is gluten-free)

PAPA GIBBONS'S SAVORY TOASTS

My father used to make these for us. They were his invention and he called them Gibbons Burgers, even though they weren't burgers, we loved them. He used white French bread, but I suggest using a healthier version of bread. I love these savory bell pepper/cheese toasts I make for lunch or dinner. They also make wonderful appetizers. Any whole-grain bread will do, but a thick piece (half of an English muffin or sliced French bread) works best. You can easily make this recipe gluten-free.

This is the recipe for one sandwich. Use these amounts for each sandwich you make.

Ingredients:

1 piece thickly sliced organic, whole-grain, sprouted-grain bread

¼ c. organic red bell pepper, washed and thinly (about ¼ inch) sliced into long strips

1–2 T. organic butter or ghee

1–2 fresh garlic organic cloves, minced

Sprinkle of unrefined sea salt (to taste)

¼ c. organic cheddar cheese (raw organic is best, vegan cheese works well too) sliced into thin (about ¼ inch) strips or grated

Directions:

1. Place bread on a baking sheet or a toaster oven rack.
2. Place bell pepper strips on bread.
3. Melt butter with garlic in it.
4. Drizzle (very lightly) melted garlic butter over bread and pepper slices.
5. Lightly sprinkle with sea salt
6. Lay slices of cheese evenly on top.
7. Place in toaster oven or oven to broil until cheese is melted.

Variation:

Substitute garlic salt for fresh garlic.

Serves one.

◆ ◆ ◆

Vegan/vegetarian/gluten-free (if gluten-free bread is used)

ROASTED VEGETABLE PITA

One summer, my son Gibbons started making these delicious sandwiches. They have become one of our favorites.

Ingredients:

1 organic, whole, sprouted-grain pita bread (gluten-free optional), warmed

½ organic zucchini, thinly sliced lengthwise

¼ c. organic red or yellow bell peppers, thinly sliced

1 organic carrot, thinly sliced

½ c. organic hummus

Directions:

1. Preheat oven to 475 degrees F.
2. Spread zucchini, peppers, and carrot slices on a roasting pan and place in oven.
3. Roast vegetables eight to10 minutes, until they are slightly soft and warm.
4. Spread hummus in the warm pita bread.
5. Lay slices of roasted vegetables in layers inside warm pita bread on top of hummus.

Variations:

Coat vegetables with a little coconut oil and sea salt before roasting for a richer and moister flavor.

Substitute grilled vegetables for roasted vegetables.

Substitute mayonnaise or sliced avocado for hummus.

Serves one.

◆ ◆ ◆

Gluten-free

LEMONY SALMON WITH DILL

Ingredients:

1 T. pure, organic coconut oil

1 organic carrots, sliced

2 organic yellow squash, sliced

4 6-oz. wild salmon steaks

¼ c. organic lemon juice

¼ c. organic ghee or butter, melted

1½ tsp. organic dill

1 tsp. organic thyme

1 organic shallot, minced

Unrefined Sea Salt to taste

Pepper to taste

Directions:

1. Preheat the oven to 400 degrees F.
2. Brush a medium baking dish with coconut oil.
3. Layer the bottom of the dish with carrots and squash.
4. Place salmon on top of vegetables.
5. In a medium bowl, combine lemon juice, butter, dill, lemon thyme, shallot, salt, and pepper.
6. Gently pour mixture over salmon.
7. Tightly cover baking dish and place in oven.
8. Bake 25–30 minutes until the salmon flakes with a fork.

Variation:

Lemon pepper makes a nice addition.

Note:

Garnish with sprigs of fresh herbs or parsley. This pairs nicely with whole-grain rice.

Serves four.

Culture and History of Food Taught to Children

Children adapt to what they are exposed to. My friend Terry French, also known as the Extreme Chef, tells how he raised his daughters as far as food was concerned:

> As far as my children and eating healthy, I have always been concerned. Fortunately they are open to lots of variety of food because they trust their dad, the Extreme Chef.
>
> My thought is always to explain the culture and history of the food presented to them, saying how children eat differently in other parts of the world. If it seemed odd to them, they are much more receptive. I use the globe and maps or google a specific place. Then they can identify what they are eating and I have them search the globe for a meal they'd like to try.
>
> I'd tell them about a child I'd met in India or Africa or Asia, explaining this was a dish they shared with me. It would open up other interesting conversation on ecology and cultural traditions.
>
> I won't say I can get them to eat sea cucumber all that quickly! But I can get a different variety of proteins and vegetables introduced when preparing Asian dishes or equatorial rice dishes. We all win on many different levels.

◆ ◆ ◆

Gluten-free

THAI COCONUT STICKY RICE WITH MANGO AND CHICKEN

My dear friend, Chef Terry French, graciously contributed this recipe for his wonderfully delicious Thai sticky rice for this book. I made this with fine grain xylitol as the sugar, and I got rave reviews!

Ingredients:

½ c. basmati rice (or ½ cup jasmine rice or ½ cup other sweet Asian rice)

14 oz. coconut milk (use the light kind if you want; it just makes it a little less rich)

½ c. sugar

1 mango (sliced)

12 oz. grilled chicken breast (cut into strips)

Directions:

1. Rice: Cook rice according to package directions, but substitute coconut milk for half of the water, and add half the sugar. It should be fairly dry when you finish cooking it, without any liquid visible in the pot.
2. Sauce: In a medium saucepan, boil the rest of the coconut milk with the second half of the sugar. Keep this at a full boil until the rice is cooked, or until it reaches a thick, syrupy consistency.
3. Presentation: Arrange the cooked coconut rice in a bowl or plate with the mango slices. Add grilled chicken breast cut into strips on top around the rice formation and dribble a bit of the sauce over the whole thing.

Serves one to two.

◆ ◆ ◆

Gluten-free

SALMON CROQUETS BY MIMI

My mother made these for us when we were growing up. My sister Mary (we all call her Myrtle) told me she frequently makes them for her family and they love them "lemony." Mary serves these warm with mashed potatoes and a spinach salad.

Ingredients:

1 can wild, red salmon (you can use fresh salmon)

5–6 whole-grain saltines (you can use a soft, whole grain, organic cracker of your choice)

1 egg (organic)

Fresh organic lemon juice to taste

Extra-virgin, organic coconut oil

Unrefined sea salt to taste

Directions:

1. Remove the bones (spine) and skin from the salmon.
2. Mush salmon, saltines, egg, and lemon juice, and form croquet. (Makes 4– 8, depending on how large you make them.)
3. Turn burner to medium heat.
4. Place about a half-inch of coconut oil in the skillet and heat coconut oil so a little drizzle of water sizzles when sprinkled onto oil.
5. Gently place croquets into oil.
6. Turn once to cook both sides until crispy and brown.
7. Remove patties from skillet to paper towel– lined plate to absorb excess oil.

Note:

These taste delicious cold the next day. They make an easy lunch to take for school or work. Serves four.

◆ ◆ ◆

Vegetarian/gluten-free

BEAN LASAGNA

This bean lasagna dish is a hearty, cost-effective meal. I love lasagna, and this is one of my family's favorite dishes.

Bake this in a 13 x 9 x 2 dish that's deep enough for the layers of the lasagna. Serve this with crusty, hot, whole-grain bread and a salad.

Ingredients:

8 oz. organic whole-grain, gluten-free, lasagna noodles
2 c. organic, sprouted great northern or pinto beans (cooked)
3 c. organic tomato sauce (preferably from a glass jar or freshly made)
2 organic, eggs
1 16-oz. container organic ricotta cheese
2 c. organic mozzarella cheese, grated
1 c. organic Parmesan cheese, grated
1 c. organic onion, chopped
1 T. extra-virgin, pure organic coconut oil
2 cloves organic garlic, minced
1 tsp. organic oregano
1 tsp. organic basil
¾ tsp. sea salt
½ tsp. black pepper

Directions:

1. Preheat oven to 375 degrees F.
2. Boil a pot of water and cook lasagna noodles until al dente. (This means they are soft, but not too soft; there is a tiny bit of hardness to them.) When they are al dente, remove from heat, drain, and set aside.
3. Beat eggs.
4. Combine eggs with ricotta cheese, mozzarella cheese, ¼ cup of the Parmesan cheese, and ½ teaspoon of the sea salt. Set aside.
5. Sauté onion in a very large skillet or heavy-bottomed pot with coconut oil until almost translucent.
6. Add cooked beans, minced garlic, remaining ¼ teaspoon of sea salt, black pepper, oregano, and basil; sauté a few more minutes.
7. Add tomato sauce and stir a few more minutes until combined well.

8. In the baking dish, layer the lasagna: Start with ⅓ of the bean-tomato mixture, followed by a layer of noodles, then half of the cheese mixture evenly. Repeat the layers. Finish with the last ⅓ of the bean-tomato mixture and sprinkle the remaining Parmesan cheese over the top.
9. Bake 30 minutes.
10. Serve warm.

Note:

I love to use roasted tomato sauce in this recipe. Muir Glen has a wonderful roasted tomato sauce that comes in a glass jar. (See Resources.) It is easy to use a whole grain, gluten-free lasagna noodle. See resources for gluten-free noodles.

Serves four to six.

◆ ◆ ◆

Vegetarian/gluten-free

BROCCOLI LASAGNA

I frequently serve this broccoli lasagna when I have company. It is easy to make ahead of time, refrigerate, and then reheat for the dinner. This looks complicated, but it's actually easy. You can buy frozen broccoli and spinach and thaw them, and buy cheeses already grated. This will make the preparation easier.

I usually make two or three lasagnas at a time and freeze them. Having them on hand makes entertaining easy. I have had many of my meat-eating friends tell me they absolutely love this lasagna, so it has passed the "non-vegetarian dinner guest test" at my home (and this is in Texas, where that test can be a tough one!).

Bake this lasagna in a 13 x 9 x 2 dish that's deep enough for the layers of the lasagna. Serve with salad and crusty, whole-grain (preferably gluten-free) bread.

Ingredients (all organic):

8 oz. organic whole-grain, gluten-free lasagna noodles
2 organic, pasture raised eggs
1 16-oz. container organic ricotta cheese
1 c. organic mozzarella cheese, grated
1 c. organic Parmesan cheese, grated
½ c. organic parsley (fresh), chopped
¼ tsp. unrefined, sea salt
¼ tsp. black pepper
1 c. organic onion, chopped
1 T. extra-virgin, pure coconut oil
1 c. organic mushrooms, sliced
2 organic cloves garlic, minced
3½ c. organic broccoli crowns, chopped
3 c. organic tomato sauce
Dash of cayenne pepper
Pinch of garlic salt
Pinch of onion powder
⅛ tsp. basil (dried)
⅛ tsp. thyme (dried)
⅛ tsp. parsley (dried)
⅛ tsp. savory (dried)
⅛ tsp. sage (dried)
1 tsp. miso
¼ c. non-chlorinated water

Directions:

1. Preheat oven to 375 degrees F.
2. Combine cayenne pepper, garlic salt, onion powder, basil, thyme, dried parsley, savory, and sage with the tomato sauce and set aside.
3. Dissolve miso in the ¼ cup of water. Set aside.

4. Boil a pot of water and cook lasagna noodles until al dente. (This means they are soft, but not too soft; there is a tiny bit of hard ness to them.) When they are al dente, remove from heat, drain, and set aside.
5. Beat eggs.
6. Combine eggs with ricotta cheese, mozzarella cheese, ¼ cup of the Parmesan cheese, and fresh parsley. Set aside.
7. Sauté onions in a large skillet with coconut oil until almost translucent, then add the mushrooms and minced garlic and sauté a few more minutes.
8. Add miso water to the skillet with onion mixture carefully, so it doesn't splatter.
9. Quickly add chopped broccoli, salt and pepper and sauté a few minutes. Remove from heat and set aside.
10. In the baking dish, layer the lasagna: Start with ⅓ of the tomato sauce, followed by a layer of noodles, then half of the cheese/egg/herb mixture evenly, then half of the vegetable mixture evenly. Repeat the layers. Finish with the last ⅓ of the tomato sauce and sprinkle the remaining Parmesan cheese over the top.
11. Bake 25 to 30 minutes.

Note:

I love to use roasted tomato sauce with this recipe. Garlic salt can be found in the spice area at the grocery store. You can also simply mince some garlic and add it to some sea salt to make your own. It is easy to use gluten-free lasagna noodles in this recipe, but you don't have to use gluten-free. For gluten-free noodles, see Resources.

Serves six to eight.

Gluten-free

CHICKEN WITH ARTICHOKES AND MUSHROOM SAUCE

Quality is important. Buy organic, humanely and pasture-raised fowl.

Ingredients:

1 c. organic artichoke hearts, chopped

8 oz. of organic chicken breast cut into 1-inch cubes.

4 c. organic sliced mushrooms (Portobello or button work well)

1½ teaspoons of pure organic, coconut oil

½ c. water

1 vegetable bouillon cube

2 T. organic chopped red onion

3 c. organic tomatoes (you can use ones from a jar) chopped into chunks

½ tsp. ground thyme (fresh is best, but dried is fine)

½ tsp. ground organic oregano (fresh is best, but dried is fine)

1 T. fresh organic parsley (minced)

Sea salt to taste (about 1 teaspoon)

Directions:

1. Melt the vegetable bouillon cube in the water and set aside for a minute.
2. Heat oil in a saucepan over medium to high heat, then sauté onion and mushrooms for about 5 minutes or until they are slightly brown.
3. Place the chicken in a broiler pan and broil about 10 minutes and then turn over and cook until they are done like you like them. (You can cook mushrooms lightly coated with coconut oil the same way and use them as vegetarian versions of this recipe for anyone who is vegetarian or vegan.) Then remove and set aside and keep it warm.

4. Add the bouillon water broth to the mushroom, onion mixture and bring to a boil.
5. When the water in the saucepan has reduced to almost half, add the tomatoes, artichokes hearts, oregano, thyme, and sea salt. Simmer for about 5 minutes. Stir frequently. When the sauce has thickened, remove from heat.
6. Add the parsley and keep warm.
7. Serve the chicken with the artichoke, mushroom sauce served over it.

Variation:

For a vegan version, you can substitute Portobello mushrooms for the chicken. Simply cook the mushrooms with the sauce, but add about a little (¼ cup) more water.

Note:

When finished cooking, simply slice the Portobello mushrooms in large ½ thick slices and serve the sauce over them.

Serves one to two.

Food for Children Over Four or Five

(or those who can handle the types of serving tools)

Gluten-free

SHISH KEBABS

Traditionally, a shish kebab (meaning roast meat) is meat cooked on a stick. The shish kebab was developed by nomadic peoples who once inhabited the area around present-day Turkey. Today variations of the dish exist in almost every culture. Asians call them satay and are usually served with a dipping sauce. The French call them brochettes, meaning skewers.

Whatever the terminology, this dish is easy to prepare, serve, and eat.

Shish kebabs make a perfect dinner whether you are entertaining, want an easy dinner at home, or when you're camping. They can be prepared in advance and assembled fairly quickly. Allow the chicken and/or mushrooms to marinate for at least an hour in the refrigerator to absorb the flavor. The marinade can be as easy as your favorite teriyaki sauce, Italian salad dressing, or barbeque sauce—or you can be creative and mix and match fruit juices, hot sauces, herbs, and spices to create your own signature marinade.

Dinner on a stick is especially fun as a hands-on cooking and eating experience for kids. The main utensil needed will be metal or wood skewers. Always soak wood skewers 20–30 minutes, and then dry off any excess water before assembling; this keeps them from catching fire while cooking. Monitor children closely when they are handling the skewers.

Mushrooms are also a wonderful, hearty substitute for meat. I have combined the two here to make a rich, hearty meal. Mix in a variety of flavors and colors by adding different fruits and vegetables. When everything comes together, you will have a beautiful, fun, and delicious meal!

Ingredients:

1 lb. organic, pasture-raised chicken, cut in 1½-inch cubes

1 lb. button organic mushrooms, stems removed

1 c. gluten-free teriyaki sauce
1 T. extra-virgin, pure coconut oil
1 large organic red onion, cut in 1 inch squares
2 organic zucchini, thickly sliced
1½ c. organic cherry tomatoes
1 fresh, organic pineapple, cored and peeled, then cut into 1-inch squares unrefined
Salt and Pepper to taste (optional)

Directions:

1. Place chicken and mushrooms in a large zip-top bag with enough teriyaki sauce to completely cover them. Refrigerate an hour or two, turning bag over every once in a while to make sure chicken and mushrooms are thoroughly marinated.
2. If you are using a grill, start the fire. (Skewers can also be broiled or baked in the oven or grilled on an electric indoor grill.)
3. If using wood skewers, soak in water 20–30 minutes, then dry.
4. Rub skewers with coconut oil.
5. Assemble skewers with chicken, mushrooms, onion, zucchini, tomatoes, and pineapple.
6. Put skewers in a large zip-top baggie with teriyaki sauce and keep in the refrigerator until time to cook.
7. Bake, broil, or grill shish kebabs over medium heat for about 10 minutes or until chicken is done to your liking. Turn the kebabs every few minutes. Watch to make sure they don't burn.
8. Season with salt and pepper to taste.
9. Serve warm. You can remove the children's food from their skewer, before they get it and be sure to monitor the children while they are handling any of the skewers.

Variation:

1. Make your own marinade for this dish. Using olive oil, garlic, herbs, soy sauce, and a little honey or brown rice syrup, you can make a tasty marinade.
2. Use any kind of meat you desire; they all work really well.
3. This is an easy dish to make vegetarian/vegan. Simply leave out the chicken. It tastes just as delicious!

Notes:

1. Teriyaki sauce is rather salty. Because of this, you may not need to add additional salt and pepper to this recipe.
2. You can assemble the skewers of chicken (meat) in advance.
3. For a nice glaze and to keep kebabs moister, brush them with marinade while cooking.
4. You can use mushrooms, tempeh, beef, bison, or turkey instead of the chicken.

This recipe fills approximately 25 8-inch skewers.

◆ ◆ ◆

Vegetarian/gluten-free

BROCCOLI QUICHE

I love to make quiche. Easy to make and store, it can be eaten warm or cold. It made a great dish to make for the children to take with them for lunch at school.

I use a variety of ingredients for the filling. This is my basic recipe using a pre-made, whole-grain, gluten-free crust from the frozen food department at my grocery store. You can easily prepare this dish for company or parties, too.

Ingredients:

1 whole-grain organic gluten-free piecrust
½ organic onion, chopped

1 tsp. extra-virgin, pure organic coconut oil

1¼ c. fresh organic broccoli crowns, cut into small pieces

1 c. organic milk (milk of choice; coconut, rice, almond all work well)

4 organic, pasture, humanely raised eggs, well beaten

1 tsp. organic parsley, dried or freshly minced (optional)

½ tsp. organic chives, dried or freshly minced (optional)

1 T. organic mustard

1 c. organic cheddar cheese, grated

½ c. organic mozzarella cheese, grated

½ tsp. unrefined sea salt

¼ tsp. pepper (optional)

Directions:

1. Preheat oven to 350 degrees F.
2. Pierce piecrust with the tines of a fork to make a few air holes in the crust, so it won't make air-filled bubbles when it is cooking.
3. Bake crust empty for about 5 minutes. Remove from oven to cool slightly.
4. Sauté onion and coconut oil in a skillet, until onion is slightly soft and translucent.
5. Add broccoli to the skillet mixture and sauté for just a moment before removing from heat.
6. Mix together milk, eggs, parsley, and chives and set aside.
7. Spread mustard evenly around the base of the piecrust.
8. Spread onions and broccoli evenly around the piecrust over mustard.
9. Combine cheeses and sprinkle over broccoli.
10. Sprinkle salt and pepper over broccoli and cheese.
11. Carefully pour milk, and egg mixture over broccoli and cheese. Do this so the mixture goes down in between the broccoli and cheese and is evenly distributed around the whole quiche.

12. Bake 30–45 minutes, until top is golden brown and the pie seems firm. (You can also stick a toothpick in the center to see if it comes out clean.)
13. Let quiche sit for at least five minutes before cutting.

Variations:

1. Substitute asparagus or baby spinach for broccoli.
2. Use different cheeses like Monterey Jack.
3. You can use vegan cheese and alternative milk in this as well.

Serves four to six.

◆ ◆ ◆

Vegan/vegetarian/gluten-free

TACO SALAD

Sometimes we like something crunchy, salty, and Mexican! Growing up in Texas meant having a true appreciation for Mexican food. You can buy healthier chips today that have whole grains or even bean flour in them. Remember, blue corn has 20 percent more protein and 8 percent less starch. Colorful food is usually healthier than less colorful options.

I make my beans and rice ahead of time and then have them ready to put together when I am ready to make this salad.

Ingredients:

2½–3 c. cooked organic, black beans (recipe p. 189)
2½–3 c. cooked organic, whole-grain brown rice (recipe p.233
1 head organic romaine lettuce
1 bunch organic cilantro, chopped
1 organic tomato, chopped
1 pack organic whole-grain, organic tortilla chips (gluten-free works well)

Directions:

1. You may want to combine these steps on each individual serving plate so each serving has a beautiful complete presentation.
2. Have black beans and rice warm and ready, set aside.
3. Tear lettuce into small, bite-sized pieces and put that and cilantro in bowl.
4. Add rice on top of lettuce.
5. Add the cooked and warm beans.
6. Sprinkle cilantro and tomato sprinkled on top.
7. Add sensational sea salt to taste.
8. Crumble a handful or two of tortilla chips on top.
9. Serve with sliced tomato.

Serves four to six.

◆ ◆ ◆

Gluten-free, vegetarian (depending on the hot dog used)

TEXAS CORNDOGS

I grew up eating corn dogs at the Texas State Fair. I had a great cornbread recipe and started making this version of the corndog. Delicious! This became one of my children's favorite meals. This cornbread recipe is one of the best! You can be made all by itself without the hot dog. If you make the cornbread, bake it in a 4 x 5 pan. I grew up eating cornbread with black eyed peas made by my mother and grandmother. That is a Texas/southern tradition. It's still one of my and my children's favorite meals.

Here is my version of a corndog. I don't add a stick to this corndog, but it tastes great, anyway. You can buy the sticks at a specialty cooking stores.

This recipe calls for tiny loaf pans made for baking bread. They are sold separately or as a large pan with individual, mini-loaf spaces. Many stores, including Sur La Table, Williams-Sonoma, Crate and Barrel, and

Target sell the pans. If you don't want to buy one, simply use a small cooking container that's about an inch and a half deep and longer than it is wide. You can also use muffin cups to put them in. They work just fine.

Blue corn has 20 percent more protein and about 8 percent less starch than yellow cornmeal. Beware: it does make your bread blue! So, in this instance, it may be more visually aesthetic to use yellow. Be sure to buy certified organic cornmeal. This recipe calls for quinoa flour and is gluten-free.

Serve these corndogs warm with a little mustard or ketchup on the side.

Ingredients:

1\. T. extra-virgin, pure organic coconut oil
1 c. whole, GMO-free organic cornmeal
½ c. whole grain, sprouted, organic teff, quinoa or coconut flour
1½ T. baking powder (non-aluminum)
½ tsp. baking soda
½ tsp. sea salt
2 organic eggs
1½ c. organic buttermilk
1 T. organic ghee, melted
2 T. organic honey (don't use honey with children under 18 months; use maple syrup instead)
1 pack organic, regular, organic hot dogs or GMO-free, organic vegetarian hot dogs (depending on your preference)

Directions:

1. Preheat oven to 450 degrees F.
2. Place coconut oil in the tiniest loaf pans you can find, and let it melt in the oven for a couple of minutes. Remove from oven and set aside.
3. Sift together cornmeal, coconut flour, baking powder, baking soda, and sea salt.
4. In a large bowl, beat eggs.
5. Add buttermilk, melted ghee, honey, and melted coconut oil to beaten eggs, and beat together.

6. Place a tiny piece of parchment paper in the bottom of each pan. Coat with coconut oil, and then turn it over and leave it in the bottom of the pan. (This will make it much easier to take out of the pan when finished.)
7. Cut hot dogs to fit into the pan lengthwise. Leave a little space at each end for the cornbread to cover it.
8. Add dry ingredients to wet ingredients.
9. Pour batter into the pans over parchment paper.
10. Place hot dogs in the center of the pan, so that they are surrounded by the corn bread on all sides.
11. Bake about 35 minutes. Tops should be golden brown and sides should have pulled away from the sides of the pan. (You can do the toothpick test to see if the center is done.)
12. Serve warm.

Notes:

1. Have hot dogs ready. When the batter is ready, it is best to get it into the pans and then the oven quickly. Larger-sized hot dogs usually taste better.
2. Make this recipe without the hot dog for a delicious Texas corn bread.
3. You can buy organic, sprouted, flours from Blue Mountain Organics. See resources.

This recipe makes about 12 mini corndogs.

◆ ◆ ◆

Vegetarian/gluten-free (if you use gluten-free tortillas)

VEGETARIAN MOO SHU-Note: this recipe contains peanuts.

This is a delicious, vegetarian version of moo shu.

Ingredients:

4–6 organic, sprouted, whole-grain tortillas

4 tsp. extra-virgin pure organic coconut oil
4 organic eggs
¼ lb. organic mushrooms
4 c. organic green cabbage, shredded
1 c. organic carrots, shredded
3 organic scallions, thinly sliced
2 T. gluten-free teriyaki sauce
¼ c. raw, organic peanuts, chopped
¼ c. hoisin sauce

Directions:

1. Preheat oven to 350 degrees F.
2. Wrap tortillas in parchment paper and then wrap in foil, so that you don't have foil touching your food.
3. Heat tortillas in oven 5 to 8 minutes, just until they are warm.
4. Heat 2 tsp. of the coconut oil in a large skillet.
5. Scramble three eggs, remove from skillet, and set aside.
6. Add remaining oil to skillet and sauté mushrooms until soft.
7. Add cabbage, carrots, scallions, and teriyaki sauce, and cook for another few minutes.
8. Beat remaining egg. Add remaining egg to mixture and sauté a few moments.
9. Add peanuts and reserved eggs to the mixture and stir.
10. Take warm tortillas out of oven.
11. Taking one tortilla at a time, spread with a generous amount of hoisin sauce and then add a large spoonful of mushroom mixture.
12. Roll up tortillas.
13. Serve warm.

Variation:

Substitute whole-grain pita bread for tortillas for more of a Middle Eastern version.

Note:

The purple cabbage is healthier because of the high antioxidant level, but it makes your food look blue when cooked. You can serve it at Halloween!

Serves four to six.

◆ ◆ ◆

Vegetarian/gluten-free (if you use gluten free bread crumbs)

EDY'S TEX-MEX STUFFED TOMATOES

My daughter–in-law makes these wonderful Texas style stuffed tomatoes all the time.

They are delicious. She makes them a little differently all the time. Sometimes she adds a pinch of cumin to the quinoa. This is her basic recipe. This recipe may be preferred by older children.

Ingredients:

2 Large tomatoes
1 cup cooked quinoa
Small can diced green chiles
1/2 tsp smoked paprika
1/4 cup shredded smoked cheddar or gouda
Sea Salt and pepper
Whole wheat bread crumbs (optional)

Directions:

1. Make quinoa according to package directions
2. Cut holes in tops of tomatoes, scoop out insides, sprinkle salt inside, turn upside down on paper towels to drain for 10 minutes.
3. Mix quinoa with green chiles, smoked paprika, shredded cheese, and sea salt and pepper to taste.
4. Pre-heat oven to 350 degrees.
5. Fill tomatoes with quinoa mixture.
6. Top with bread crumbs if desired

7. Bake for 15 minutes or until heated through

Serves 2

Note:

Soak the quinoa for 18 hours in non-chlorinated water before cooking to remove phytic acid.

◆ ◆ ◆

Vegan/vegetarian/gluten-free

MARY'S SPAGHETTI SQUASH WITH MARINARA

My sister Mary cooked spaghetti squash for her children when they were growing up. They didn't know this was different from the spaghetti everyone else was eating. She'd simply add vegetables to this dish and her children loved it.

Ingredients:

2 organic whole spaghetti squash

¼ cup pure, organic coconut oil

Sea salt to taste

4 cups prepared (jarred) marinara sauce (Seeds of Change, Eden Foods or Whole Foods have a good variety to choose from.)

1 organic zucchini (chopped into small chunks)

Directions:

1. Preheat the oven to 450 degrees F.

2. Cut squashes in half and scrape out seeds with a large spoon. Coat the spaghetti squash with coconut oil and sprinkle with sea salt.

3. Place flesh side down in a large casserole dish or baking sheet and roast for 30 to 40 minutes until fully cooked.

4. Remove from the oven and let rest until cool enough to handle.

5. Heat a tablespoon of coconut oil in a large saucepan or frying pan and sauté the zucchini until tender.

6. Add the marinara sauce to the frying pan and heat until warm.

7. When squash is cool, scrape the large spaghetti strands out of the spaghetti squash.

8. Place the spaghetti squash in the pan with the warm marinara and combine until spaghetti squash is hot and well mixed.

9. Serve warm and enjoy.

Notes:

1. You can add vegetables such as broccoli florets and cook with the zucchini for a more vegetable-filled dish.
2. This might seem like a side dish to some people.

Variation:

Add a garnish of Parmesan cheese to this dish.

Serves four to six.

Side Dishes

Vegan/vegetarian/gluten-free

BLACK-EYED PEAS

Black-eyed peas make a wonderful high-protein meal. I grew up in Texas where black-eyed peas and cornbread make up a traditional meal. Leftovers of this meal freeze well. Start this recipe the day before you want to serve it.

Ingredients:

- 2 c. organic black-eyed peas
- 1 piece kombu seaweed
- 1 tsp. extra-virgin, pure coconut oil
- ½ c. organic onion, chopped
- ½ tsp. pure, unrefined sea salt

Directions:

1. Soak black-eyed peas 18 hours or overnight in purified water.
2. Discard soaking water.
3. Put black-eyed peas in a large pot and add enough water to cover peas plus an additional inch. Bring to a boil.
4. Drain water.
5. Add enough new water to the pot to cover the peas by about an inch. Add seaweed, oil, onion, sea salt, and black pepper.
6. Bring to a boil, then reduce heat and simmer 30–45 minutes or until the beans are soft.
7. Serve slightly warm.

Notes:

1. For a baby food or a small child, place about a cup of this finished food in the blender with a few tablespoons of alternative milk such as unsweetened coconut milk and blend until creamy.

2. If you don't have time to soak black-eyed peas overnight, you will have to cook them a little longer.
3. Kombu seaweed can usually be found in the Asian foods area of Whole Foods Market, as well as other stores. Buy certified organic seaweed. Seaweed contributes many nutrients to any recipe and helps break down the enzymes in beans and peas so they are more easily digested. You can discard the seaweed after cooking or eat it. I add it to almost all of my soups and beans when I am cooking them. There are a variety of seaweeds to choose from. They all have a variety of nutrients in them. Flavors vary. Experiment!
4. Make the cornbread (only) from the corn dog recipe and serve it with this recipe. It's delicious!

Variation:

1. You can use any bean or pea to cook with this recipe.
2. For a sweeter flavor, add a drop or two of barbeque sauce. When I do this, I serve it on New Year's Day for good luck!

Note:

1. This might seem like a side dish to some people.
2. Soaking the peas helps remove the phytic acid in the peas.

Serves two to three.

◆ ◆ ◆

Vegan/vegetarian/gluten-free

ROASTED POTATOES WITH ROSEMARY

Potatoes and rosemary go well together. I grow rosemary in my yard and love to add it to my dishes. This easy recipe has a rich flavor that tastes comforting on a cold day. Note that the term "new potatoes" and "red potatoes" refer to the same potato. If you have never tried them, you're in for a treat. They loved it when I made purple potatoes and had friends over for dinner.

Ingredients:

4 large organic purple, Yukon gold, or sweet potatoes cut in 2-inch chunks

2 T. organic sweet red onion, finely chopped

1 small organic cloves garlic, freshly minced

1 T. fresh organic rosemary (finely chopped)

3 T. extra-virgin pure coconut oil, slightly melted

Whole sea salt to taste pepper to taste

1 T. organic extra-virgin olive oil

Directions:

1. Preheat oven to 350 degrees F.
2. Combine potatoes, onion, garlic, rosemary, coconut oil, salt, and pepper in a large baking dish. Make sure potatoes are coated well.
3. Bake 30 minutes, stir, and bake another 30 minutes.
4. Remove potatoes from oven, place in another dish, and toss with olive oil.

Notes:

1. For a baby food or a smaller child, place about a cup of the finished food in the blender or food processor with 3-4 T. water or unsweetened milk and blend until creamy and smooth.
2. You can melt coconut oil in the pan while it is preheating. This will make the oil easier to mix with the other ingredients. It will also coat the baking pan well.
3. To chop rosemary, remove leaves from stem and then chop leaves.

Serves four, depending on the size of the potatoes.

Vegan/vegetarian/gluten-free

SWEET POTATO FRIES

I make sweet potato fries as a nutritious and easy snack in the afternoon (perfect for children right out of school) or as a side dish. I love easy baking recipes because the dish can cook while I am busy doing other things. This really satisfies your sweet and salty cravings.

The sweet potato is actually from the morning glory family, and it's packed with vitamin A and beta-carotene. This high-fiber food adds color and variety to a meal with its beautiful blend of sweet and tart flavors.

You can have your children rub the oil and sea salt on the potatoes. They will eat a wider variety of healthy food if you involve them in the preparation process. Tell them they are chefs or scientific researchers.

My daughter likes to make these super thin so they'll get crisp.

Ingredients:

2–3 organic sweet potatoes, washed well

2 T. extra-virgin, pure organic coconut oil

1–2 tsp. unrefined sea salt

Directions:

1. Preheat oven to 400 degrees F.
2. Slice potatoes thinly (about ¼ of an inch thick) or slice into wedges. The thinner the wedge, the crispier it will get and the quicker it will cook.
3. Rub with coconut oil and sprinkle with sea salt.
4. Lay slices or wedges out on a large, flat, coconut oiled baking dish with low sides.
5. Bake until they are soft enough to put a fork into easily. (The time will depend on the thickness of the slices, maybe 25 to 40 minutes.)

6. After they are baked, place under the broiler for another 4 minutes or so to get them a browner and crispier. Taste test them carefully; you can judge how long it takes with your oven.

Notes:

1. For a baby food or a small child, place about a cup of this finished food in the blender with a few tablespoons of alternative milk such as unsweetened coconut milk and blend until creamy.
2. These taste best fresh, so only make as many as you will eat right away. Adjust the recipe accordingly.
3. This dish makes a great treat for your dog.
4. This might seem like a side dish to some people.

Serves one person per potato.

◆ ◆ ◆

Vegetarian/gluten-free

APPLE-CRANBERRIES SWEET POTATOES

Ingredients:

5 organic sweet potatoes, peeled and cut in 1-inch chunks
2 T. organic ghee or butter
1 large organic green apple, cored, peeled, and diced
1 c. raw organic cranberries
½ c. organic raisins
1 T. xylitol
½ c. organic orange juice

Directions:

1. Preheat oven to 350 degrees F.
2. Place sweet potatoes in a large, buttered baking dish, and top with apples, cranberries, ghee and raisins.
3. Sprinkle xylitol over it all.
4. Pour orange juice over top.

5. Cover and bake for 1 hour and 15 minutes, or until sweet potatoes are tender when pierced with a fork.

Notes:

For a baby food or a smaller child, place about a cup of the finished food in the blender or food processor with about 3-4 unsweetened nut milk and blend until creamy. This recipe stores easily in the refrigerator or freezer.

This might seem like a side dish to some people.

Variations:

1. Substitute yams for sweet potatoes.
2. Add ¼ cup chopped pecans or walnuts.
3. Substitute dried cranberries for fresh.

Serves four to six.

◆ ◆ ◆

Vegan/vegetarian/gluten-free

SWISS CHARD WITH SAUTÉED MUSHROOMS

I love to make this recipe whenever I have Swiss chard fresh from my garden. It makes a great side dish, or a quick and easy vegetarian main dish. Shitake mushrooms are a great choice for this recipe, but you can use any variety.

Ingredients:

1 bunch organic Swiss chard, washed
1 T. extra-virgin, pure, organic coconut oil
1 T. organic ghee or butter (optional: use a little more coconut oil if you are vegan and don't want to use ghee or butter)
¼ c. organic red onion, chopped
2 c. organic mushrooms, brushed, rinsed, and sliced
3 T. warm, non-chlorinated water
1 T. miso

1 tsp. organic garlic, minced
Unrefined sea salt

Directions:

1. Stack Swiss chard leaves, roll them up, and cut crossways into strips.
2. Set Swiss chard aside.
3. Melt coconut oil and ghee or butter in a large skillet over medium heat. Add onion and sauté 1–2 minutes.
4. Add mushrooms and sauté until onion gets a little clear and soft, about 3–4 minutes.
5. Mix warm water and miso until miso makes a broth.
6. Add miso broth to skillet and incorporate.
7. Add Swiss chard to skillet and sauté lightly until it is bright green and wilts. (This takes only a few minutes.)
8. Add garlic, salt, and sauté lightly for a few seconds.
9. Remove from heat.

Notes:

1. For a baby food or a small child, place about a cup of this mixture and a few sprigs of parsley in the food processor or blender with a few tablespoons of alternative milk such as unsweetened coconut milk. Blend until creamy.
2. Add more onion if you love onions.
3. Add a little more water or oil if onions seem too dry while you're sautéing them.
4. This might seem like a side dish to some people.

Serves four to six.

Vegan/vegetarian/gluten-free

WHOLE-GRAIN RICE WITH BOUILLON

Coconut oil, ghee, sea salt, and bouillon cube add more richness and flavor to a basic rice dish. If the bouillon cube has salt in it, do not add additional salt.

Ingredients:

2 c. organic whole-grain brown basmati rice

41/2 c. water

¼ tsp. sea salt (optional)

1 T. extra-virgin pure organic coconut oil (optional)

1–2 vegetable bouillon cubes, dissolved in the water

1–2 T. organic ghee (optional)

Directions:

1. Soak rice 18 hours in pure, non-chlorinated water to remove the phytic acid. Rinse rice thoroughly in a small-weave sieve until water runs clear. Set aside.
2. Bring water to a boil in a large pot. Add rice, sea salt, if using, coconut oil, if using, and bouillon cube(s), and let boil for a couple of minutes while stirring.
3. Reduce heat to a simmer.
4. Cover pot tightly and do not disturb for 35 to 40 minutes. Do not stir.
5. When it looks as if all the water is absorbed, rice is ready.
6. Let rice sit in the pot but off the heat about 5 minutes. Fluff rice with a fork.
7. Add ghee, if using, and stir gently.
8. Gently scoop out the rice and serve warm.

Notes:

1. For a baby food or a small child, place about a cup of this finished food in the blender with a few tablespoons of alternative

milk such as unsweetened coconut milk. Blend until creamy.

2. Long-grain rice is fluffier than medium grain, which is a little moister.
3. This might seem like a side dish to some people.

Variations:

1. Add a little sautéed onion to this after cooking for a richer and different flavor.
2. Add some raisins and pine nuts for a different sweet and nutty flavor.
3. Substitute whole-grain quinoa for rice. (It will cook in about half the time.)

Note:

I frequently soak my rice and lentils overnight to sprout them. This makes them easier to digest after cooking. I drain off the water and then use new water for cooking. When I need a little less water in which to cook them in, because they are softer. So, if you soak your lentils and rice overnight (which I recommend), pour off the water you soak them in and then use about 2 cups of fresh water for cooking. When you cook it, just make sure there is about1/2 inch of water over the rice/lentil mixture when you start to cook it.

Serves four to six.

◆ ◆ ◆

egetarian/gluten-free

SAUTÉED ASPARAGUS

Although we eat asparagus raw a good deal of the time, this lightly sautéed recipe is delicious. Serve this dish warm.

Ingredients:

2 lb. organic asparagus

1 T. extra-virgin pure organic coconut oil

1 T. organic ghee

Whole, unrefined, sea salt to taste

Pepper to taste

½ c. organic Parmesan cheese (optional)

Directions:

1. Rinse asparagus and trim off thick, harder ends. Cut asparagus into 1½–inch pieces.
2. Sauté asparagus and coconut oil in a skillet or wok about 5 minutes over medium heat until it becomes bright green and is just warm.
3. Add ghee quickly and let it melt as you sauté one more minute and sprinkle with salt and pepper.
4. Remove from heat.
5. Sprinkle Parmesan cheese, if using, on top. Serve slightly warm.

Notes:

For a baby food or a small child, place about a cup of this finished food in the blender with a few tablespoons of alternative milk such as unsweetened coconut milk or structured water. Blend until creamy. You can also add ¼ pitted, peeled avocado for extra nutrients.

Variation:

Use a mayonnaise and lemon juice sauce instead of olive oil.

Serves two to four.

◆ ◆ ◆

Vegan/vegetarian/gluten-free

BRUSSELS SPROUTS WITH CHESTNUTS

Chestnuts are low in fat and high in protein and fiber. Brussels sprouts are packed with vitamins and fiber, with only about 25 calories per half-cup. Being a member of the disease-fighting cabbage family, Brussels sprouts are also rich in phytochemicals that may protect us from cancer.

You can enjoy this delicious, healthy, and hearty dish any time, but it's especially good during the cold fall and winter months.

Ingredients:

1 c. organic chestnuts
4 c. organic Brussels sprouts
2 T. extra-virgin pure organic coconut oil
1 organic shallot, finely chopped
6 c. vegetable broth
1 T. organic ghee or butter
Sea salt to taste
Pepper to taste

Directions to cook chestnuts:

1. Using a small sharp knife, cut a cross at the bottom of each chestnut.
2. In a saucepan, bring 3 cups water to a boil. Gently drop in chestnuts using a slotted spoon, and boil about 8 minutes. (Use enough water to cover all of the chestnuts generously.)
3. Remove pan from heat and remove nuts a few at a time using a slotted spoon.
4. Gently remove the outer skin with a knife and peel off the inner skin.
5. Empty saucepan, put nuts and enough vegetable broth to just cover nuts, and put pan back on the heat.
6. Simmer about 15 minutes.
7. Drain nuts and set aside.

Directions to cook Brussels sprouts and finish:

1. Rinse and remove a few of the outer leaves of Brussels sprouts that might be yellow or wilted. (You can cut off the root end carefully to leave Brussels sprouts intact.)

2. In a heavy frying pan that has a lid, melt coconut oil and add shallot. Sauté the mixture for a few minutes until shallot is soft.
3. Add Brussels sprouts and enough vegetable broth to barely cover the sprouts. Cover and simmer on medium heat, stirring occasionally, about 10 minutes.
4. Add chestnuts, stir, cover, and cook until Brussels sprouts and chestnuts are tender, about 5 minutes.
5. Stir in ghee (or butter), salt, and pepper.
6. Serve warm to anyone with good chewing ability, but puree in a blender until smooth, if the child has a few or no teeth.

Note:

For a baby food or a smaller child, place about a cup of the finished food in the food processor with about 3 T. unsweetened non-dairy milk and process until creamy. You can also add ¼ a pitted, peeled avocado to make this more nutrient dense.

Serves four to six.

◆ ◆ ◆

Vegan/vegetarian/gluten-free

QUINOA

Quinoa is a complete protein, gluten-free seed that is used today as if it is a grain. It is easy to cook and has a wonderful nutty flavor. Quinoa contains lysine, vitamin E, folate, magnesium, phosphorus, and manganese. There are different varieties of quinoa. The darker colored quinoa has more antioxidants because antioxidants are the color (pigment) of food.

Store quinoa in the refrigerator or freezer to avoid rancidity.

Ingredients:

1 c. organic quinoa

2 c. water

¼ tsp. sea salt

½ tsp. organic coconut oil

Directions:

1. If the quinoa is not sprouted, soak quinoa18 hours in pure, non -chlorinated water to remove the phytic acid.
2. Drain water and place quinoa in a large pot that has a good top.
3. Add the water, sea salt and coconut oil.
4. Bring to a boil, turn down the heat to simmer, cover with the top and simmer for about 15 minutes.
5. Remove quinoa from the heat and let it sit for a few minutes with the top still on it.
6. Fluff up the quinoa with a fork and serve warm.

Note:

1. For a baby food, simply place the quinoa and a little bit of water or milk of choice in a blender . Blend until creamy.
2. I like to have quinoa with stir-fried vegetables or steamed broccoli. I also enjoy it as a side dish or breakfast dish.
3. Soaking the quinoa (a seed) in water helps remove the phytic acid. If you want to do it more completely, add 1 tsp. of whey to the 18 hour soaking water.

Serves two to three.

◆ ◆ ◆

Vegan/vegetarian/gluten-free

BASIC WHOLE GRAIN RICE

Ingredients:

1 c. organic whole grain rice

1 T. organic coconut oil

2 c. pure water

1 tsp. unrefined sea salt

1 large piece of organic kombu seaweed

Directions:

1. Soak the rice for 18 hours or overnight in pure water to sprout it, then pour off the water and get fresh water to cook it in. You won't need to cook it quite as long if you have soaked it all night. You would only take about 20 minutes.)
2. Place the coconut oil, sea salt, seaweed, rice in a large saucepan.
3. Add water (2 cups) to pan.
4. Bring to a boil over high heat.
5. Reduce heat to medium and cover with a lid. Allow liquid to be absorbed (about 40 minutes). When only a few bubbles remain on the surface, reduce heat to a minimum, cover tightly, and steam about 10 minutes without stirring.
6. You can remove the seaweed if desired.
7. Serve warm.

Note:

1. For a baby food, simply place the rice and a little bit of water or milk in a blender. You can also add 1 T. finely minced fresh parsley or one-fourth an avocado (pitted and peeled). Blend until creamy.
2. Soaking the rice in water helps remove the phytic acid. If you want to do it more completely, add 1 tsp. of whey to the 18 hour soaking water.

Serves three to four.

◆ ◆ ◆

Vegan/vegetarian/gluten-free

BROWN RICE AND CASHEWS

Ingredients:

2 c. organic whole long-grain rice

4 c. water

¾–1 c. organic cashews

2 T. organic sweet onion, finely chopped

1 tsp. pure, unrefined coconut oil

Whole sea salt (Nancy's sensational sea salt seasoning) to taste

Directions:

1. Soak the rice for 18 hours or overnight in pure, non-chlorinated water to sprout it, then pour off the water and get fresh water to cook it in. You won't need to cook it quite as long if you have soaked it all night. You would only take about 20 minutes.)
2. Soak the cashews18 hours or overnight in pure, non-chlorinated water to remove the phytic acid.
3. Place rice, water, onion, pinch of the sea salt, coconut oil and cashews into a large pot.
4. Bring rice to a boil and stir for a few moments.
5. Reduce heat to low, cover with a tight-fitting lid, and simmer without stirring about 40 minutes.
6. Fluff rice with a fork and leave it in the pot, off of heat, about 5 to 10 minutes. (This will give you drier, fluffier rice.)
7. Sea salt to taste.

Notes:

1. For a baby food or a small child, place about a cup of this finished food in the blender with a few tablespoons of alternative milk such as coconut milk. Blend until creamy.
2. While it is still warm, you can also place the rice cashew mixture in a wood bowl, cover with a warm dishtowel, and let sit a few minutes.
3. Soaking the rice and nuts in water helps remove the phytic acid. If you want to do it more completely, add 1 tsp. of whey to the 18 hour soaking water.

Vegetarian/gluten-free (if using gluten free bread crumbs)

BAKED SQUASH CASSEROLE

This recipe tastes great in the fall or winter. You can use yellow crook-necked squash or zucchini squash.

Ingredients:

1½ T. organic extra-virgin, pure coconut oil

2 ½ lb. organic zucchini squash (or crookneck squash) cut into 1" chunks

1 c. organic cottage cheese

1 c. (3-4 ounces) organic Monterey Jack cheese, grated.

2 organic eggs, beaten

¾ tsp. dill seeds

½ tsp. unrefined sea salt

1 T. organic butter (cut up into little bits)

½ c. whole grain, organic, dry breadcrumbs

Directions:

1. Preheat oven to 350 degrees F.
2. Place squash in salted water and cook at a simmer for about 5 minutes.
3. Drain the squash well.
4. Grease a large casserole dish with coconut oil.
5. Combine squash, cottage cheese, grated cheese, beaten eggs, dill seeds, and unrefined sea salt and place in the casserole dish.
6. Bake the casserole, in the preheated oven, uncovered for 15 minutes.
7. Remove the casserole and sprinkle the breadcrumbs over the top of the squash mixture, and dot it with the butter.
8. Bake the casserole for another 10 to 15 minutes.

Note:

You can actually make baby food out of this recipe by simply putting a little bit in the blender with a little unsweetened milk and blend until creamy.

Serves four to six.

Sandwiches, Pizzas, Burgers, and Flatbread

Vegetarian/gluten-free (if gluten-free bread is used)

TOASTY CHEESE SANDWICH

When my children were growing up, Toasty Cheese Sandwiches were one of their favorite things. I used a sandwich toaster griddle, but you can use a skillet and something heavy to press the sandwich down when it is cooking. My children liked it with only cheese until they got a little older.

This tastes great served with a small cup of tomato soup.

Ingredients:

Butter (or ghee) or mayonnaise (optional)
2 slices organic sprouted, whole-grain bread
2 thin slices organic cheddar cheese (vegan cheese can be used)
1 organic tomato slice (optional)
Extra-virgin, organic coconut oil

Directions:

1. Spread a tiny bit of butter or mayonnaise on a slice of bread (if using).
2. Place one slice of cheese on bread, and top with tomato (if using), and other cheese slice.
3. Top with other bread slice.
4. Melt a tiny bit of coconut oil in a frying pan and place sandwich in pan. (I used a sandwich toaster/press from William Sonoma.)
5. Cook until down side is a toasty brown.
6. Gently turn over sandwich and cook the other side until is toasty brown.
7. Slice on a diagonal.

Variation:

Substitute your favorite cheese for cheddar.

Makes one sandwich.

Vegetarian/gluten-free (if gluten-free bread is used)

◆ ◆ ◆

SPINACH AND BLACK BEAN FLATBREAD OR PIZZA

This is a slight variation of a recipe made by my niece Claire and her husband. Theirs is a little spicier. They add salsa to it as a garnish.

Ingredients:

- 1 10-oz. organic, sprouted, whole-grain pizza flatbread or gluten-free pizza crust
- 1 c. cooked organic black beans (about one can)
- ⅓ c. minced organic onion
- 1 tsp. ground cumin
- 1 garlic clove, minced
- ½ c. fresh or bottled organic tomato pasta sauce
- 1 c. frozen or fresh organic spinach (if using frozen, thaw and dry it first and if using fresh, tear into bite size pieces)
- ½ c. organic Monterey Jack cheese, grated
- ½ c. organic sharp cheddar, grated

Directions:

1. Preheat oven to 375 degrees F.
2. Place pizza crust on a baking sheet; bake 5 minutes or until crisp.
3. Mash beans with a fork; combine beans, onion, cumin, and garlic in a medium bowl, stirring to combine.
4. Spread bean mixture over crust, leaving a 1-inch border.
5. Spoon pasta sauce evenly over bean mixture; top with spinach.

6. Sprinkle with cheeses.
7. Bake 15 minutes or until crust is lightly browned.

Variations:

1. Use vegan cheese instead.
2. Brush coconut oil on crust and sprinkle freshly grated Parmesan cheese before toasting in a 450-degree oven for 5 to 7 minutes.

Serves two to four

◆ ◆ ◆

Vegetarian/gluten-free (if gluten-free bread is used)

PORTOBELLO MUSHROOM BURGER

This Portobello Mushroom Burger is one of my family's favorite savory meals. I have made this for many non-vegetarian Texans with success, much to their surprise! This was a favorite meal of Larry Hagman (J. R. Ewing in the TV show *Dallas*) that I made for him. The quantities here are enough for one person. You can make as many sandwiches as you want by adjusting the ingredient amounts.

Ingredients:

1 large organic portobello mushroom
1 T. gluten-free soy sauce (Nama Shoyu is the brand I use)
1 organic, sprouted, whole-grain hamburger bun or whole grain bread
¼ c. organic goat cheese, sliced

Directions:

1. Brush off mushroom and remove stem.
2. Soak in soy sauce at least five minutes (20 minutes is better).
3. Bake the mushroom with the soy sauce at 350 degrees F. or broil

in an oven, just until thoroughly warm, making sure it is moist with the soy sauce.

4. Warmed or toasted bun.
5. Place cheese on top of mushroom and leave in oven a couple of minutes until the cheese is soft.
6. Remove mushroom from oven and place on bun.
7. Place top bun on sandwich.
8. Serve warm.

Variations:

1. Add avocado slices instead of the goat cheese for a nondairy version.
2. Add healthy mayonnaise.

Note:

Udi's has a gluten-free bun. My favorite, which is not gluten-free, is made by Alvarado Bakery. (See Resources.)

Serves one.

◆ ◆ ◆

Vegetarian/gluten-free (if gluten-free bread is used)

QUICK AND EASY PIZZA

This Quick and Easy Pizza makes a great lunch, dinner, or after-school snack. Enjoy! It uses truffle oil, one of my favorite oils for recipes. It makes dishes rich and taste unique.

Ingredients:

1 organic, sprouted whole-grain, ready-to-use pizza crust or flatbread

1½ c. shredded organic mozzarella cheese

½ c. organic tomatoes, thinly sliced (¼-inch thick

1 organic clove garlic, minced

¼ c. red or sweet organic onion, thinly sliced

Few leaves basil (fresh), chopped

½ tsp. truffle oil (optional)

Directions:

1. Preheat oven to 375 degrees F.
2. Place half of cheese evenly on the top of the pizza crust or bread.
3. Spread tomatoes evenly on top
4. Put garlic, onion, and basil evenly on top of the tomatoes.
5. Lightly sprinkle remaining cheese over the pizza.
6. Drizzle truffle oil, if using, over the top for an extra-special taste!
7. Place pizza in oven until crust is baked, or the cheese is melted and slightly brown on the edges.

Variation:

Use a whole-grain pita, an English muffin, or simply a thick slice of whole-grain bread instead of pizza crust. Adjust ingredient amounts as needed.

Serves two.

◆ ◆ ◆

Vegan/vegetarian/gluten-free (if gluten-free bread is used)

PITA SANDWICH

I like many different kinds of pita sandwiches, but this is an all-time satisfying one. When you use avocado, it is best to eat the pita sandwich right away. If you won't be eating this right away, wrap it tightly to keep the air out, or the avocado can turn dark. Because of the nature of avocado, you can mash the avocado with a little lemon juice to help it stay fresher and greener longer. You can also buy gluten-free pita bread.

Ingredients:

1 sprouted, whole-grain, organic pita

1 organic avocado, sliced

¼ c. organic black beans, cooked 1 small, organic tomato, chopped

3 T. organic sprouts

Pinch of sea salt

1–2 slices organic mozzarella cheese (optional if you wish it to be vegan)

Directions:

Layer ingredients in pita bread. Enjoy!

Variations:

1. Substitute goat cheese for mozzarella.
2. Add some chopped onion.
3. Add a few leaves of spinach.
4. Substitute kidney beans for black beans.
5. Substitute hummus, mustard or mayonnaise for avocado.

Serves one.

◆ ◆ ◆

Vegan/vegetarian/gluten-free (if gluten-free bread is used)

HUMMUS SANDWICH

This Hummus Sandwich is one of my favorites! I like to make this when I'm in a confined place with little resources.

Ingredients:

½ c. organic hummus

2 slices organic, soft, sprouted, whole-grain bread of choice

Directions:

1. Spread some hummus on each slice of bread.
2. Cover with the other piece of bread.
3. Slice into two halves.

Serves one.

Vegan/vegetarian/gluten-free (if gluten-free bread is used)

AVOCADO SPROUT SANDWICH

I have been enjoying this yummy sandwich since I was a teenager. In fact, I grew up eating sprout and butter sandwiches. Today, I prefer to use avocado instead of the butter.

You can wrap this tightly if you take this sandwich with you, or you can eat it right away. If you don't eat immediately, put it in the refrigerator until you are ready.

Ingredients:

1 organic avocado
2 slices organic, soft, sprouted, whole-grain bread of choice
Sea salt
½–1 c. sprouts of choice (alfalfa, broccoli, etc.)

Directions:

1. Mash avocado until creamy.
2. Spread some avocado on each slice of bread.
3. Sprinkle with sea salt.
4. Heap sprouts on top of avocado.
5. Cover with the other piece of bread.

Serves one.

Salads

Vegan/vegetarian/gluten-free

HEARTY BEAN SALAD

My daughter Amanda creates wonderful recipes. This Hearty Been Salad is one of her best. It is high in protein, has great flavor, and can be a complete meal.

Ingredients:

2 c. cooked organic black beans

2 T. organic extra-virgin olive oil

1 c. chopped organic cucumber

2 c. organic baby kale or baby romaine greens (torn into bite-size pieces)

1 organic avocado, sliced

1 clove minced organic garlic

¼ c. chopped organic cilantro

Sea salt to taste

Pepper to taste

Directions:

1. Warm up black beans.
2. Combine warm beans, olive oil, cucumber, kale, avocado, garlic, and cilantro. Stir well.
3. Season with salt and pepper to taste.

Serves two.

Vegan/vegetarian/raw/gluten-free

SPINACH SALAD

This easy-to-make Spinach Salad recipe even pleases people who usually don't usually like salads. It was one of my son's favorites growing up. The fresh vitamin C in the citrus fruit helps the body absorb the iron in the spinach better.

Ingredients:

1 bunch baby organic spinach (fresh)

1 c. raw organic almond slivers

2 organic tangerines or oranges peeled, seeded and sectioned

½ c. sprouts

Poppy seed dressing (recipe below)

Directions:

1. Tear spinach into bite sized pieces.
2. Add all ingredients and toss with Poppy Seed Dressing.
3. Top with some more sprouts.

Serves two to four.

◆ ◆ ◆

Vegetarian/gluten-free

POPPY SEED DRESSING

Directions:

2 T. lemon juice

2 T. apple cider vinegar

2 T. poppy seeds

3 T. maple syrup

⅛ tsp. unrefined sea salt

3 T. sunflower seed oil

2/3 c. plain or vanilla or coconut organic yogurt

Directions:

Mix lemon juice, vinegar, maple syrup, poppy seeds, and sea salt together until the maple syrup is dissolved well. Then stir in sunflower seed oil and yogurt.

Note: This dressing can be refrigerated for up to a week.

◆ ◆ ◆

Vegan/vegetarian/raw/gluten-free

RED CABBAGE SLAW

Ingredients:

1 head organic cabbage
4 organic apples (Granny Smith or tart apples work well)
2 organic carrots
1 cup organic raisins
2 T. organic apple cider vinegar
1 T. xylitol
Dash of Nancy's Sensational sea salt seasoning (or unrefined sea salt)

Directions:

1. Soak the raisins in a little water to make them soft and plump.
2. Dissolve xylitol in apple cider vinegar.
3. Grate the cabbage, apples, and carrots.
4. Combine all ingredients in a bowl.
5. Eat at room temperature or refrigerate and serve chilled. Sometimes it tastes better after sitting overnight. The flavors get melded together.

Variation:

Add a few tablespoons of a healthy version of mayonnaise for a richer creamier dish.

Serves four to six.

Vegan/vegetarian/raw/gluten-free

◆ ◆ ◆

GRANNY'S CARROT RAISIN SALAD

I love Granny's Carrot Raisin Salad. It always reminds me of my childhood spent at my grandmother's home. When I make this salad, I make a double recipe to have it handy for easy snacks or a part of meals throughout the week. I leave the peel on the carrots because they are full of nutrients.

Ingredients:

1 bag organic carrots, grated
1–2 c. organic raisins
¼ c. mayonnaise

Directions:

1. Mix all ingredients together and enjoy!

Variation:

Substitute ¼ cup orange juice mixed with 2 tablespoons raw, organic, extra-virgin, pure coconut oil for mayonnaise.

Serves four, depending on serving size.

Vegan/vegetarian/gluten-free (depending on the pita bread)

MIDDLE EASTERN BEAN SALAD WITH PITA BREAD

Many people say they just get tired of eating salads. This Middle Eastern Bean Salad has flavor and provides an alternative to a basic garden salad. It makes a great lunch to take to school or work.

Ingredients:

1½ c. cooked organic pinto, kidney, or black beans
2 organic scallions, finely chopped
1 c. organic cucumber, chopped
¼ c. organic red bell pepper, chopped
1 small clove organic garlic, minced
¼ c. organic lemon juice (fresh)
4 T. organic extra-virgin olive oil
4 T. organic pine nuts (pre soaked for 18 hours in pure water and dehydrated or dried)
¼ tsp. organic oregano
½ tsp. organic parsley
½ T. organic dill (fresh)
½ tsp. sea salt
4 c. organic romaine lettuce, chopped
Sprouted, whole-grain, organic pita chips preferably, gluten-free (optional)

Directions:

1. In a large bowl, combine beans, scallions, cucumber, red bell pepper, garlic, lemon juice, olive oil, pine nuts, oregano, parsley, dill, and sea salt. Let sit at least 15–20 minutes and allow the juices to meld together.
2. Toss the bean/cucumber mixture with the romaine lettuce right before serving so the lettuce doesn't get soggy.
3. Serve with whole grain gluten-free pita bread or pita chips.

Serves four, depending on serving size.

Vegan/vegetarian/raw/gluten-free

YUMMY SEED AND BROCCOLI SALAD

This salad is a favorite. If you have any left over, it tastes excellent the next day. It is also makes a super salad for lunch on the go.

Salad Ingredients:

10 c. bite-sized organic broccoli crowns
1 c. organic, raw, sprouted sunflower seeds
1 c. organic, raw, sprouted pumpkin seeds
1 c. organic dates, chopped or raisins
¾ c. organic red onion, chopped finely

Dressing Ingredients:

1 c. organic milk of choice
1 organic avocado
4 T. organic apple cider vinegar
¾ tsp. sea salt
¼ c. organic, extra-virgin olive oil
3 T. raw, unrefined organic honey (don't use honey with children under 18 months; use maple syrup instead)

Directions:

1. Combine all salad ingredients in a large bowl and set aside.
2. Combine all dressing ingredients in a blender and blend.
3. Combine dressing with salad ingredients in the large bowl, and toss well.
4. Let it sit in the refrigerator for at least an hour before serving. The ingredients need to meld together for a symphony of flavor.

Variation:

Substitute raisins or currants for dates.

Notes:

1. Each cup of broccoli serves one person. Total recipe serves ten.
2. You can purchases organic, raw, sprouted seeds from Go Raw or Blue Mountain Organics (See Resources).
3. You can sprout raw, organic seeds yourself by soaking them in pure water for 18 hours. Add a little whey to the soaking water to help remove the phytic acid more completely. Then dry the seeds by placing them in a dehydrator or in a low heat warmer.

◆ ◆ ◆

Vegan/vegetarian/raw/gluten-free

SUZIE HUMPHREYS'S GREEK SALAD

My friend Suzie makes the best Greek salad. She generously gave me her recipe.

Ingredients:

1 c. organic romaine lettuce, torn in bite-sized pieces
1 organic cucumber, peeled, seeded, and chopped
1 organic red pepper, seeded and chopped
¼ c. organic red onion, cut into small, thin silvers
¼ c. organic black olives
¼ c. organic green onions
1 stalk organic celery, chopped
1 organic tomato, chopped
¾ c. feta cheese (raw, organic, and with vegetable enzymes)
La Martinique salad dressing

Directions:

Toss all ingredients together with salad dressing.

Variation:

Substitute another vinaigrette dressing for La Martinique dressing.

Snack Foods

Some of the best snacks are simply fresh fruits and vegetables cut up into bite sized pieces. I frequently take raw, freshly washed green beans or raw okra and rub or sprinkle unrefined sea salt on them. They make a great snack! Green beans have an insulin-type of effect on the body, so they make particularly good snacks for anyone who has to regulate their blood sugar.

Place about a half of a cup in small snack containers or zip lock baggies. That way, you can then grab them quickly throughout the week for quick snacks. They taste delicious.

Vegan/vegetarian/gluten-free

HOMEMADE HUMMUS

This is a basic recipe you can use as a guide to creating your own magical hummus. It goes well with whole grain, gluten-free crackers, chips, cut up veggies (example: red bell pepper or sliced cucumber), pita chips, etc. I use it as my sandwich spread for many things. I even make hummus sandwiches with it. It is a delicious high protein staple to keep around for emergency snacks or meals.

Ingredients:

2 c. cooked organic chickpeas

¼ c. organic tahini

2-3 organic garlic cloves (minced)

2 T. fresh organic lemon juice

½ tsp. unrefined sea salt

1 T. freshly chopped organic parsley (or 1 tsp. dried)

¼ tsp. cumin (you may want to add more of this spice depending on your own personal taste.)

¼ tsp. paprika (optional)

¼ c. organic cashew butter (optional; I love the extra rich flavor)

Directions:

1. Combine all ingredients in a food processor and blend until creamy.
2. Serve at room temperature as a dip or spread.
3. I like to serve this on tomato slices and yellow bell pepper slices.
4. Store in the refrigerator in a tightly sealed container. If sealed well, it will keep almost a week.

Note:

My sister Liz grates carrots to add to various meals (e.g., pasta sauces) for more veggies in the diet. You can add them to this too.

◆ ◆ ◆

Vegan/vegetarian/raw/gluten-free

GUACAMOLE

I'm from Texas and I love to eat guacamole. I use it as a dip or sandwich spread. I always make it fresh and use it immediately. One of the reasons I like this dip is the avocado. An avocado is a kind of perfect food. The avocado is a great source of potassium, Vitamin K, B, C and E. One avocado has around 4 grams of protein. The avocado is also a great source of monounsaturated fat, which is considered a good fat.

I estimate ½ an avocado per person.

Ingredients:

3-4 avocados, peeled, pitted and mashed.

1 small tomato chopped

1 tsp. sweet red onion, finely grated

¼ cup chopped cilantro

1 T. fresh lemon juice

½ tsp. Sensational Sea Salt Seasoning or unrefined sea salt

Directions:

1. Mix all ingredients together well.
2. Serve with healthy, organic cut up veggies (like sliced cucumber or red bell pepper) as the dipping chips or multi grain, organic gluten free tortilla chips.

Note:

If you are not using immediately, place in container and put a piece of wax paper over the top and seal it in a way that will not allow air to touch the surface. Store in refrigerator in an airtight container. Will keep about 1 day.

Serves 6-8

◆ ◆ ◆

Vegan/vegetarian/raw/gluten-free

TRAIL MIX

I had trouble finding a trail mix that I liked that didn't have some sort of sugar added to it, so I decided to make my own. Trail mix is wonderful to keep as a snack for traveling, as daily running-around emergency food, or as a snack at the office or school.

You can purchase organic, sprouted nuts and seeds online from Blue Mountain Organics or Go Raw (See resources). If you do that you won't need to soak the seeds and nuts, because they will already have the phytic acid removed from them.

This recipe needs to be started a couple of days before you need it and is best if you can use a dehydrator to dry the nuts. Soaking the nuts, or sprouting them, removes the phytic acid and also makes them easier to chew. This is a raw recipe, but you can use your own version of nuts. If you love chocolate, add it to this mix and it will meld right in! If you just want a hint of cacao, use cacao powder instead of cacao nibs.

Ingredients:

½ c. organic, raw pecans
½ c. organic, raw pine nuts
½ c. organic, raw almonds
½ c. organic, raw walnuts
½ c. organic, raw pistachios
½ c. organic, raw brazil nuts
½ c. organic, raw pumpkin seeds
½ c. organic, raw sunflower seeds
½ c. coconut (fresh or dried), shredded
½ c. organic, raw apricots (unsweetened, non-sulfured and dried), chopped
1 c. organic, raw cherries (unsweetened and dried), chopped
½ c. organic, raw raisins
½ c. organic, raw medjool dates (pitted and chopped)
½ c. organic, raw papaya (unsweetened and dried), chopped
¼ tsp. sea salt

Directions:

1. Soak all (raw, non-sprouted) nuts 18 hours in pure (non-chlorinated) water, and then let them dry well.
2. Dry them in a dehydrator for a few hours, if you have one. If you don't, spread them on a cookie sheet and let them sit in a very dry, slightly warm oven (less than 118 degrees F.) at least an hour.
3. Combine all ingredients in a bowl.
4. Make sure that any child who eats this trail mix, chews slowly and really well.

Notes:

1. Soaking the nuts makes them more digestible and helps eliminate the phytic acid and enzyme inhibitors.
2. Store this in an airtight glass container, or put it into small

containers ready to grab quickly. Keep it in the refrigerator, so it will stay fresh longer.

3. Eat this mixture within a week. Since the nuts are soaked, they won't last as long. You can freeze it and then thaw out what you need.

Makes 7 cups.

◆ ◆ ◆

Vegan/vegetarian/raw/gluten-free

ENERGY PROTEIN BARS

These are really healthy, easy, and delicious! The natural sugar content of raisins and dates is high; but the remainder consists of protein, fat and mineral products. I like to use them in this recipe for the flavor and the health benefits. Raisins and dates are both a good source of carbohydrates for energy.

Dates contain copper, sulphur, iron, magnesium, and fluoric acid. They are an excellent source of potassium.[123] Raisins are also rich in B vitamins, iron, and potassium. This might seem surprising, but "compounds found in raisins fight bacteria in the mouth that cause cavities and gum disease," according to research presented today at the 105th General Meeting of the American Society of Microbiology.[124] I made this type of food as a desert for my children.

Ingredients:

1 cup organic raisins

½ c. organic almonds, soaked at least 12–18 hours in water. Discard the soaking water.

4 organic medjool dates, pitted and soaked at least 1 hour in a little bit of water. Save the water. Add at least two tablespoons of this water to the food-processing mixture.

2 T. date soaking water or plain water

¼ c. freshly ground organic flax seeds

½ dropper of liquid stevia (plain or toffee flavor)

2 c. organic steel cut, sprouted oats (gluten-free)

4 T. raw, organic sprouted sunflower seeds and/or pumpkin seeds or a mixture of both.

1 c. vanilla flavored organic protein powder of your choice (I use Garden of Life Protein Powder.)

1tsp. sprouted, apricot seed butter (optional)

¼ tsp. sea salt

1 T. extra-virgin, pure, organic coconut oil

Directions:

1. Combine all ingredients in a food processor and pulse the mixture until it creates a dough-like consistency. If it's too thick, add a little more water. If it's too thin, add a little more oats until it is thicker.
2. Line a 2-inch-deep glass or ceramic baking dish with wax paper, and then spread out the mixture in the baking dish about 1⁄2-inch thick. Depending on the size of your dish, you may need two dishes. You can put wax paper or plastic wrap over the mixture and use it to press the bars flat.
3. Place in refrigerator for at least an hour to firm. If you want it firmer, place it in the freezer.
4. Using the wax paper, lift the bars out of the dish and place them on a cutting board. Remove the wax paper and slice into bars.

Notes:

1. Soaking almonds makes them easier to digest.
2. Store bars in an airtight container wrapped in plastic wrap or parchment paper. Store in the refrigerator for added freshness.

3. Oats are naturally gluten-free, but they must be stored and transported in gluten-free containers for them to be labeled gluten-free.
4. You can purchase raw, sprouted gluten-free oats, sprouted seeds, and sprouted seed butter from Blue Mountain Organics.

◆ ◆ ◆

Vegan/vegetarian/raw/gluten-free

KALE CHIPS

This delicious, nutritious, and easy snack or side dish is made with a dehydrator, but you can use an oven on a very low temperature instead. Kale chips are crispy, thin chips made from fresh kale. Kale shrinks a great deal, so make one bunch for each person. This is a fun and easy recipe that the children can help make. The mesquite and cinnamon are optional.

Ingredients:

1 bunch fresh organic kale per person
Organic pure coconut oil (about 1 T.)
Sea salt (about ¼ tsp.)
Mesquite powder (about ¼ tsp.)
Ceylon cinnamon (about ¼ tsp.)

Directions:

1. Cut kale in approximately 2-inch-square pieces.
2. Rub each piece with coconut oil.
3. Sprinkle lightly with all of the seasonings.
4. Dehydrate about 5 to 10 hours until crispy.

Notes:

1. These chips are very fragile, so I usually make them during the day while I am able to watch them.

2. Store kale chips in an airtight container so they will keep for a few days.
3. I sometimes make this as a desert. I drizzle the tiniest bit of honey or maple syrup on my kale chips before dehydrating. It makes them sweet as well as spicy and salty. A tiny bit rubbed into the mix works well.

◆ ◆ ◆

Vegetarian/gluten-free

MUSHROOM NIBBLES

I love mushrooms and make these quick-and-easy Mushroom Nibbles all the time. I serve them for lunch or a snack. They also make terrific as appetizers and/or a side dish, especially when served warm.

Ingredients:

10 or more button or small cap organic mushrooms

Enough soy sauce (organic and unpasteurized) to cover the mushrooms

2 T. organic pesto

¼ c. raw, organic goat cheese

Directions:

1. Brush off mushrooms and remove stems.
2. Soak mushrooms in soy sauce two hours or overnight.
3. After soaking, place mushrooms in a baking dish.
4. Fill mushrooms with goat cheese and top with a dab of pesto.
5. Warm mushrooms in an oven, toaster oven, or warming drawer.
6. Serve slightly warm.

Note:

Soak the stems, too, chop them, and save them for use in other recipes.

When warming, keep the temperature under 118 degrees F. to keep the enzymes alive.

Vegan/vegetarian/raw/gluten-free

NORI ROLLS WITH NUT PÂTÉ

The first time I made this recipe was when I needed a quick lunch to take on an airplane. This is great finger food for lunch boxes, snacks to take along and makes a terrific appetizer. Get the children to make this with you. When children help make the food they are more likely to try it and like it!

Ingredients:

2–3 nori sheets

1 c. Nut Pâté (following recipe)

1–2 organic avocados, sliced

1 organic carrot, julienne

½ c. organic sprouts (sunflower or broccoli)

½ c. soy sauce (gluten-free, unpasteurized, organic; for dipping)

Directions:

1. Lay out nori sheets (shiny side down) on a flat surface or a bamboo (sushi) mat (that can roll up).
2. Spread a thick layer of Nut Pâté on a middle section of each nori sheet all the way across, about an inch tall, leaving about a half-inch border from the outside edge.
3. Spread slices of avocado over Nut Pâté, staying inside the edge by about a half-inch. Lay them horizontally.
4. Place carrots in a thick layer on the sheets in a horizontal position from you.
5. Lay an even layer of sprouts across the carrots and avocado.
6. Take the end of the nori sheet right in front of you and start rolling it, away from you.
7. Seal the final edge with a little water to make it stick.
8. Slice this across the roll into about 1-inch-thick rolls.
9. Dip pieces in soy sauce and enjoy.

Notes:

1. The nori will cut easier if you use a very sharp knife.
2. Avocado is one of the two main ingredients in the recipe, so use a half or a whole avocado for each roll.
3. You can substitute hummus for the nut pate.

◆ ◆ ◆

Vegan/vegetarian/raw/gluten-free

NUT PÂTÉ

This is an easy, rich, and savory snack or appetizer. I use this as a filling for my Nori Rolls with Nut Pâté. You could also serve this with crackers or with slices of vegetables as a dip. It is delicious as a filling for celery.

Ingredients:

½ c. organic walnuts, soaked 12 to 18 hours, if they aren't already sprouted, (pour off water and dry nuts before using- either a food dehydrator or in a low-heat food warmer)

1½ c. organic pecans, soaked 12 to 18 hours, if they aren't already sprouted (pour off water and dry nuts before using either a food dehydrator or in a low-heat food warmer)

1 organic red bell pepper, chopped

2 stalks organic celery, chopped

2 T. organic lemon or lime juice (fresh)

1 tsp. unrefined sea salt or Nancy's Sensational Sea Salt Seasoning

Dash of mesquite powder (optional)

Directions:

1. Combine all ingredients in a food processor.
2. Add a little water if necessary. Process until creamy.
3. Store in a well-sealed container in the refrigerator.

Note:

This can keep for about four days refrigerated.

Vegan/vegetarian/raw/gluten-free

ANTS ON A LOG

This easy favorite has been around since I was a little girl. My sister Liz suggested I add this to the book.

Ingredients:

Organic peanut butter or a nut butter of your choice

Organic celery sticks cut into 2- to 3-inch lengths.

Raisins

Directions:

1. Spread peanut or a variation on the celery sticks.
2. Place raisins in a line down the peanut butter.

Variation:

Add a tiny bit of sprouted apricot seed butter to the butter mixture for added nutritional benefits.

Notes:

1. You can purchase organic, raw, sprouted, nut and seed butters from Blue Mountain Organics.
2. Almond butter and even sunflower seed butter work fine with this recipe.

◆ ◆ ◆

Vegan/vegetarian/raw/gluten-free

ANNIE'S APPLE SNACKS

I grew up eating apples with peanut butter on them. My nephew's wife uses sunflower seed butter for her daughter Annie who is allergic to peanuts. The Blue Mountain Organics Sprouted Nut Butters or Sunbutter works great with this snack.

Ingredients:

1 organic apple
Organic nut or seed butter of choice

Directions:

1. Core apple then make slices of the apple in crescent shaped slices about ¼ of an inch thick.
2. Spread peanut butter, almond butter, or seed butter over each slice and then put another slice of apple on top to make an apple-butter sandwich.

◆ ◆ ◆

Vegan/vegetarian/raw/gluten-free

ISHY'S APPLE CITRUS SNACK

Ingredients:

1 organic apple (cored and seeded and freshly, sliced into crescent moon shape slices)
1 organic orange
1 organic lemon

Directions:

1. Squeeze the orange and lemon juice into a container.
2. Place the apple slices in a ziplock baggie.
3. Pour juice into the bag and close it up.
4. Refrigerate for a few hours or more.

Bread

Vegetarian/gluten-free

NANCY'S CORNBREAD

I grew up eating cornbread and black-eyed peas. I love this combination. The cornbread I developed when my children were young became part of my children's favorite meals—and still is today. If you are into jalapeno peppers and your children are old enough for spicy food, you can add them chopped up in this bread for a little Texas kick!

Blue corn has 20 percent more protein and about 8 percent less starch than yellow cornmeal. Beware: it does make your bread blue, so you may find it more visually aesthetic to use the yellow variety. Be sure to buy certified organic cornmeal.

This recipe also calls for gluten-free quinoa, oatmeal, or teff flour as the other flour.

Ingredients:

1. T. extra-virgin, pure, organic coconut oil
1 c. whole, non-GMO organic cornmeal
½ c. whole grain, sprouted organic quinoa, gluten-free oatmeal or teff flour
1½ T. baking powder (non-aluminum)
½ tsp. baking soda
½ tsp. unrefined sea salt
2 organic, pasture raised eggs
1½ c. organic buttermilk
1 T. organic ghee, melted
2 T. raw unrefined organic honey (don't use honey with children under 18 months; use maple syrup instead)

Directions:

1. Preheat oven to 450 degrees F.
2. Place coconut oil in a 4x5 loaf pan or wrought iron skillet, and let it melt in the oven for a couple of minutes. Remove from oven and set aside.
3. Sift together cornmeal, quinoa flour, baking powder, baking soda, and sea salt.
4. In a large bowl, beat eggs.
5. Add buttermilk, melted ghee, honey, and melted coconut oil to beaten eggs, and beat together.
6. Place a tiny piece of parchment paper in the bottom of the pan, but you don't need to if it's a wrought iron skillet. Coat with coconut oil, and then turn it over and leave it in the bottom of the pan. (This will make it much easier to take out of the pan when finished.)
7. Add dry ingredients to wet ingredients.
8. Pour batter into the pans over parchment paper.
9. Bake about 35 minutes. Tops should be golden brown and sides should have pulled away from the sides of the pan. (You can do the toothpick test to see if the center is done.)
10. Serve warm.

Note:

Blue mountain organics sells sprouted, organic flours.

Desserts

Popsicles

Ideally, we shouldn't consume desert or teach our children to eat them either, but here are a few versions of deserts that may be healthier that other choices.

These special treats are wonderful in the summer on a hot day. It is easy to make healthy homemade variations of a popsicle. You can use infused mint water or if you have a blender, you can make up a fruit. If you choose to create your own fruit pop, be careful about the color of fruit you choose because some of them—blueberry and cherry, for example—can stain clothing.

The only thing you need is really good fruit that you like.

A pound of fruit will yield two to three servings of popsicles. You can juice fruits and vegetables and use them in your popsicles as well. I like using the whole fruit, because then it contains the fiber and the fiber helps slow down the natural sugars as they enter the blood stream.

For someone who needs more nutritional impact or calories in his or her diet, add to the mixture a teaspoon or two of raw, extra-virgin, pure coconut oil or coconut oil with the coconut meat in it or a teaspoon of maca root powder or chia seeds. These can boost the nutritional impact of the sorbet without noticeably changing the flavor.

Here are two recipes you can use as guidelines for creating your own Popsicle delights. I love to use strawberries best, but the red fruits can stain clothing. So, you may want to use fruits that don't stain.

Vegan/vegetarian/raw/gluten-free

MANGO POPSICLES

Ingredients:

1½ c. organic mango (peeled, pitted)

½ c. pure water

Pinch of sea salt (optional)

Directions:

1. Blend all ingredients in food processor until smooth and creamy.
2. Place in a molds and place in freezer until firm.

Variation:

You can use any of your favorite fruit for this pop.

◆ ◆ ◆

Vegan/vegetarian/raw/gluten-free

PEACH POPSICLES

Ingredients:

1 lb. organic peaches, peeled, pitted, and sliced

1 c. pure mineral rich water

Juice of one orange

Directions:

1. Blend all ingredients in food processor until smooth and creamy.
2. Place in a mold and place in freezer until firm.

Note:

You can use the peach peel, but it looks "prettier" without the peel.

Puddings

Vegetarian/gluten-free

COOL BLUEBERRY TAPIOCA DESSERT

Ingredients:

1 whole organic egg

2 c. organic coconut milk (vanilla, unsweetened)

¼ c. organic tapioca

½ tsp. vanilla extract

2 tsp. xylitol

1 c. organic blueberries

Directions:

1. Wisk eggs together with milk, tapioca, vanilla, and xylitol and put in a saucepan. Heat and stir until the mixture thickens.
2. Remove from heat and put in a mixing bowl.
3. Stir in blueberries, reserving a few to use as garnish on the top of each one.
4. Pour the mixture into 4 serving dishes trying to put equal amounts of blueberries in each dish. Top with remaining blueberries.
5. Refrigerate for about 20 minutes.
6. Serve when the tapioca is firm.

Serves four.

Variation:

1. You can substitute any berry or cherry for the blueberries in this recipe.
2. Add a drop or two of stevia if you want it sweeter.

Vegan/vegetarian/raw/gluten-free

CHOCOLATE PUDDING

Chocolate pudding is one of my favorite desserts. I made this for my mother and she loved it. She even made it for her music club meeting luncheon for dessert.

Chocolate is the number one antioxidant food in the world—the superfood of superfoods. It was widely used by the Mayan and Aztec cultures in their food. When the Spanish arrived in North America, they learned of it and took it back to Europe with them.

Cacao was used to treat fatigue, fever, and nervous disorders, as well as a stimulant. The bean itself is extremely healthy; it's what's added that can make the cacao unhealthy. The cacao bean is a dark purplish color and can be bitter in flavor. This is one of the reasons so much sugar is added to make sweet chocolate.

Serve this Chocolate Pudding chilled with a dollop of flavored Cashew Crème.

Ingredients:

5 organic dates, pitted and soaked in water overnight (save the water for thinning the pudding if necessary)
1 T. organic maple syrup (pure)
½ tsp. vanilla
2 organic avocados, pitted and peeled
⅓ c. organic cacao powder, raw and pure
¼ tsp. unrefined, sea salt
⅓ c. organic vanilla milk (coconut, rice, or quinoa)

Note:

For a sweeter version, add a ½ dropper of stevia liquid.

Directions:

1. Blend all ingredients in food processor until creamy.
2. Add more of the date soaking water or milk as necessary. (You want a creamy, thick, and smooth consistency.)

3. Pour pudding into individual dishes or containers.
4. Refrigerate at least 1 hour.
5. Serve with a dollop of cashew crème (or another type of crème topping) on top.

Serves three.

Cookies

Vegetarian/gluten-free

CHOCOLATE CHIP COOKIES

This recipe of chocolate chip cookies is from my book with Maryann De Leo, *Alive and Cooking.* She made these for her nephews who ate every one and wondered when she would make more. They are so delicious; I had to put them in this book.

The high protein flour and xylitol makes them a healthy alternative to regular flour/regular sugar-made cookies. The recipe calls for either raw sugar or xylitol, but I use fine grain xylitol every time I bake.

Ingredients:

1 c. pure, extra-virgin, organic coconut oil
6 T. unsweetened organic applesauce
2 T. pure vanilla extract
1¼ c. fine grain xylitol (or raw sugar)
2 c. organic, sprouted garbanzo bean flour
1 tsp. baking soda
1 tsp. unrefined sea salt
1½ tsp. xanthan gum
1 c. organic bittersweet chocolate chips

Directions:

1. Preheat the oven to 325 degrees F. Line baking sheets with non -aluminum paper.
2. In a large bowl, mix oil, applesauce (or smashed sweet potato),

vanilla, and sugar together well.

3. In a medium bowl, sift together flour, baking soda, sea salt, and xanthan gum.
4. Using a rubber spatula, slowly add dry ingredients to the wet mixture, and stir until grainy dough is formed.
5. Fold in the chocolate chips until they are evenly distributed.
6. Using a teaspoon, scoop cookie dough onto the prepared baking pans. Space them about an inch apart. Using a fork, gently press cookies down slightly.
7. Bake cookies in the center rack for about 15 minutes. Check the bottom of a cookie to see if it is lightly brown. When the bottoms are lightly brown, they are ready.
8. Take cookies out of the oven and let cool for about 10 minutes, and then transfer each cookie to a cooking rack to cool completely.
9. Store the cookies in an airtight container at room temperature for up to three days.

Note:

Blue mountain organics sells organic, sprouted, raw garbanzo bean flour. See resources.

◆ ◆ ◆

Vegan/vegetarian/raw/gluten-free

FRUIT COOKIES

I used to make these unbaked cookies in college and have adjusted the recipe over the years. I didn't know what "raw food" was then, but I was doing raw food without knowing it. Start preparing these cookies a night ahead of time so the fruit and nuts can be thoroughly softened by the time you're ready to make them. They are easy to chew and can satisfy a sweet tooth.

You can keep cookies in the refrigerator for four to five days, or freeze them.

Ingredients:

5–6 organic figs (fresh or dried)
1 c. organic raisins
2 c. organic, sprouted sunflower seeds
2 c. organic walnuts
1 c. purified water (from soaking ingredients overnight)
1 c. organic pineapple chunks (fresh)
1 c. organic mango chunks (fresh)
2 T. pure, organic maple syrup
1 c. organic, sprouted, raw almond butter (seed or nut butter of choice)
1 tsp. organic, extra-virgin, pure coconut oil
¼ tsp. sea salt
½ c. organic fruit juice (fresh)
1 c. organic coconut (shredded)

Directions:

1. Soak figs and raisins in one bowl, for about an hour. Soak the sunflower seeds and walnuts in a separate bowl (nuts and seeds for18 hours) overnight in purified water. You can then dry the nuts or seeds by placing them in a dehydrator or a warm oven. (Soaking them helps remove the phytic acid.)
2. Retain at least 1cup of water from figs and raisins to add to the recipe.
3. Discard all of the water used for soaking the nuts and seeds. Retain only one cup of the water used for soaking the figs and raisins.
4. Blend all ingredients except shredded coconut in a food processor.
5. Using a teaspoon, scoop dough and roll into balls.
6. Roll balls in shredded coconut.

7. Place cookies on a dish and gently flatten.
8. Store in an airtight container.

Notes:

1. Sprouted nuts and seeds have a more vibrant nutritional value.
2. Good juice choices for this recipe are fresh papaya, apple, pear, and peach.
3. Using the soaking water in the recipe makes the cookie sweeter and less watery, as the water is sweeter.
4. You can order sprouted seeds, nuts, nut and seed butters from Blue Mountain Organics (see resources).

Variations:

1. If you want a more traditional cookie and you have a dehydrator, place cookies on the flat sheets and dehydrate under 115 degrees F. for about 4 hours or longer until they are easy to eat and have the consistency you desire.
2. Substitute peanut butter for almond butter.
3. Substitute dates for raisins.
4. For extra nutrition, add a teaspoon of bee pollen, lecithin, kelp, and maca root powder, or even a little raw protein powder.

◆ ◆ ◆

Vegetarian/raw/gluten-free

GLUTEN-FREE COOKIE BALLS

This cookie ball is a great alternative to a traditional sugar-laden cookies. It's only for children over 18 months of age because it contains honey.

Ingredients:

1½ c. rolled, gluten-free organic, sprouted oats

¾ c. organic , sprouted nut or seed butter of choice

⅓ c. raw, unfiltered organic honey (for children under 18 months, use maple syrup)

1 c. raw organic coconut flakes

½ c. freshly ground organic, sprouted hemp seeds

1 tsp. organic vanilla extract

¼ tsp. sea salt

Directions:

1. Combine all ingredients in a large bowl.
2. Place in the refrigerator until firm.
3. Using a teaspoon to dip out the dough, roll each teaspoon size amount into a ball. Add more nut or seed butter if the balls are too crumbly.
4. Place balls into glass containers. You can put wax paper between the layers to keep them from sticking together.
5. Store in tightly sealed containers in refrigerator for up to a week.

Variation:

For a sweeter version, chocolate chips can be added to this. Use ¼ cup of the tiny ones. Store them in an airtight container in the refrigerator.

Note:

You can order a raw, sprouted nut and seed butter, seeds and nuts from Blue Mountain Organics. See resources.

LINDA GRAY'S FAVORITE FAMILY RECIPES

Linda Gray, one of my dear friends, makes the most delicious, healthy drinks and food. She raised her children with loving care and healthy food and gave me some of her favorite recipes that she makes for her grandson. I am so excited about her sharing these marvelous recipes with you! Here are her special recipes for almond milk, green smoothie, watermelon, mint refreshing drink, and papaya custard.

Linda said, "I love to make my own almond milk and the kids love it, too! I soak the raw almonds overnight, rinse them in the morning, throw them in the Vitamix with water in the morning, and then put it all through a seed bag. The kids especially love this; it's like milking a cow. I then put it into the blender with a few handfuls of baby spinach, a scoop of protein powder (e.g., Warrior Vegan vanilla protein or Hemp protein powder), berries, a banana, or any fruit they like. I add a few ice cubes, whirl it, and voila! My kids can't believe they are consuming spinach. Yay!

"In the summer, they love to cut up watermelon, toss it in the Vitamix (or any kind of juicer), and mix it. I pour the mixture into a clear glass and add a piece of mint picked from our garden.

"We also make papaya custard. I cut up one ripe papaya (seeded and peeled) and place the pieces into the Vitamix. To that I add three whole eggs, two tablespoons of raw honey, and two tablespoons of softened butter. It whirl it, put it into individual glass containers, and refrigerate. The liquid turns into a custard, and we eat it right from the refrigerator. Yummy!"

CHAPTER 16

The Importance of Chiropractic Care

I was diagnosed with scoliosis many years ago and decided to heal it naturally as much as I could. I have had marvelous transitions to a healthier spine by having chiropractors adjust me on a regular basis. This made a big difference, along with massage therapy, ballet class, and core-strengthening exercises.

I've included this chapter written by Michael W. Hall, DC, FIACN, who has expressed well the value of chiropractic care for our children.

◆ ◆ ◆

Kids are our most precious gift! Any parent will confirm this statement. While many challenges that come with raising children, none surpass the joy that comes with having your children crawl into your lap and whisper in your ear "I love you" as they lay their head down and fall asleep. Many a night, my wife will experiences her fingers falling asleep, achiness in her back and neck, and generalized fatigue from not moving or changing positions while one of our children quietly sleeps away the night. Sacrifices come with having children—sacrifices parents endure with the hope their children will grow strong in mind and body, strong enough to face and overcome life's adversities.

Where role does chiropractic care play in raising healthy children? Chiropractors believe a healthy nervous system is the key to a healthy life. Optimal expression of the perfection within is what any parent wants of their children. Chiropractic care seeks to remove any interference in the spine and nervous system that can reduce a child's innate potential to fully express life. Chiropractors refer to these interferences as "subluxation."

Children can incur spinal subluxations in everyday events like playing, falling, sleeping in an awkward position, reading, studying, watching too much TV, and eating poorly. Spinal subluxations are simple misalignments of the vertebrae of the spine. These subluxations alter the normal transmission of neural impulses to and from the nervous system to all of our limbs and organs. Any subluxation can affect how the nervous system processes information about that limb or organ and how it would normally function. Subluxations can affect how we digest food, how our muscles contract, and, most importantly, how our brains grow and develop.

Chiropractic care seeks to remove spinal subluxations through adjustments given to the misaligned vertebra. Then chiropractors observe neurological function periodically to ensure that function is appropriate and the child is developing properly, meeting milestones of growth development and language acquisition. Children cannot always articulate pain they feel, but with gentle palpation and observation of key functions, movements, and behaviors, the chiropractor can assess and determine the need for spinal adjustments.

My wife and I regularly experience the stresses and joys of being parents of five children. We receive regular chiropractic care so we may be healthy and free of subluxation. This is just one way we model healthy behaviors for our children.

We take time together, over meals, to share, laugh, and work through things we may be dealing with, things deserving the focused attention of everyone at the table. If we are at a loss for conversation topics, we use a deck of cards in the center of the table. The cards contain questions we each answer and discuss—questions prompting deeper thought, insights, and creative solutions. It doesn't take long before we're engaged in deep conversation or a belly-aching laugh fest!

As parents, we also understand the importance of modeling an active physical lifestyle and good eating habits. We make time for family walks, bike riding, and playing catch. We minimize junk food in our diet. While it seems impossible to keep sugar completely out of a childs' diet, parents can model how to enjoy an occasional nutritious dessert free from toxic food additives, artificial sweeteners, and colorings.

To many, chiropractic care is much more than just a way to reduce spinal aches and pains. It is a lifestyle, a way of embracing all that life has to offer, all the highs and lows. Most importantly, it focuses on loving each other: lifting each other up when we are down, inspiring and encouraging each other to accomplish more than we thought possible, and working to be better today than we were yesterday.

Life will throw us many curve balls, but it will also give us opportunities and fortune. Children give us a chance to focus on how life should be and what it means to love, to put down our own agendas and stresses, to put others before ourselves, and to take care of ourselves so we can better take care of others. After all, who hasn't had his or her heart melted by a child's hug, with little fingers reaching around us and pulling us in? Can't we all do more with a hug from a child every day? Can't they do more with a regular hug from us? Go ahead, give it a try.

◆ ◆ ◆

About the Author: Michael W. Hall, DC, FIACN, has provided family-based chiropractic services in the DFW metroplex for more than 20 years. A professor of neurology, he is also director of the Functional Neurology Center at Life University. He is an accomplished international speaker on pediatrics, concussion injuries, functional neurology, and scientific advances in chiropractic care. He is a Fellow of the International Academy of Chiropractic Neurology and a Diplomat of the American Board of Chiropractic Neurology.

See details of Dr. Hall's practice (with his wife Dr. Cara Hall) listed in Resources. I have been going to him for many years.

The more that you read, the more things you will know.
The more that you learn, the more places you'll go!

—Dr. Seuss

CHAPTER 17

Exercise and Other Key Lifestyle Choices

Having a healthy lifestyle means sometimes we need to get our body moving! Exercise gets the body oxygenated and helps the lymphatic system keep moving as well as draining. The lymphatic system is part of the immune system. It is comprised of a network called lymphatic vessels. These vessels, similar to blood vessels, carry a clear fluid called lymph. These vessels carry the lymphatic fluids toward the heart. While the heart pumps the blood, it is circulated throughout the body and is cleansed by the kidneys. The lymphatic system doesn't have a pump to help it keep moving. The lymphatic system moves through the body in an upward system through the body and extremities and up toward the neck, where it enters the subclavian veins and becomes part of the plasma and blood stream once more. The lymph nodes along the way are where the lymph is filtered or cleansed. When any part of this system gets clogged, it can cause inflammation. Inflammation leads to disease.

I read the book *Dressed to Kill: The Link Between Breast Cancer and Bras* about 15 years ago. Written by medical anthropologist Sydney Singer and her assistant Soma Grismaijer, it talks about the lymphatic system and how constrictive clothing (like bras and belts) and a lack of exercise could be causing various types of cancer and disease by creating sluggish or clogged lymph nodes. Humans have three times as much lymphatic fluid as blood, making it a critical part of our health.

Signs of a compromised or clogged lymphatic system include swollen hands or feet, painful swelling of the lymph nodes, any type of arthritis or bronchitis, lack of energy or mental clarity, trouble sleeping, cysts or fibrous tumors, an inability to recover quickly from viral infections, or, last but not least, cancer.

Exercise so that the body's lymphatic system is able to stay clog-free. The movements of muscles stimulate the flow of the lymphatic system. Jumping on a rebounder or a trampoline is good, movements like running and playing are so important to a child's health. For mom, dad, or a child, lymphatic massages are helpful, especially if you feel you have clogged lymph nodes, but exercise that keeps the body moving and the lymphatic system draining is the easiest way to keep this system healthy and clog free on a regular basis. Try to do something you enjoy. Don't let exercise be a chore. Make it fun and let it lift your spirits.

Sleep and Rest

Sleep can become a problem, especially after you have a baby and you are woken up at various times of the night. It can be difficult getting enough deep sleep. You are always listening for the baby to wake. It can leave you feeling exhausted at times.

As we get older, we don't produce as much melatonin, which is what helps us sleep. If we don't have enough melatonin, our body will pull it from our serotonin reserve in order to make it. You can buy melatonin as a supplement at the store. It comes in different strengths (one to three milligrams). Dr. Gary Massad has researched melatonin and sleep problems in depth. He told me that the studies show that if you take half a milligram of melatonin around three in the afternoon and then another half gram again about an hour before bedtime, it will work most effectively.

If a melatonin supplement is taken, then it saves the store of serotonin, which affects our mood. If you aren't draining it, you will have more serotonin to help with positive moods. Melatonin works much better with ample vitamin B in your system. If you are concerned about vitamin B—if you are a vegan or vegetarian—take a good whole-food vitamin B supplement. Some think that a vitamin B spray under the tongue is the best type of supplement source, because it is absorbed better and faster. Other hormone imbalances can also disrupt our sleep patterns, so have your doctor check you for any hormone imbalance or a vitamin deficiency. I recommend only using a vitamin from a whole food source. I do not recommend ever taking synthetic vitamins.

You might also llisten to recorded sounds of rain or ocean waves to help with sleep. They can relax your mind. Experiment to find out what works best for you. In fact, what works for you might change from time to time.

What Can Help You Sleep?

1. Eat a light, comforting early supper.
2. Exercise and breathe deeply.
3. Make the bedroom a place of peace and tranquility, with as little radiation, annoying noise, and light as possible.
4. Write down your list of things you must do tomorrow. This will get all those thoughts out of your brain about the next day.
5. Think calming thoughts that are positive, uplifting, and filled with gratitude and thankfulness for 20 minutes right before bedtime.
6. Write down five things that you are grateful for, or five miracles that happened to you or your child today, or five things that you want to happen tomorrow. Focus on the most positive things you can. (I found this was a perfect time for me to put these in my children's baby books for them for the future, so they read about what they were doing as they grew up. First words, steps, discoveries, accomplishments, food favorites, people they met, funny events, and more.)
7. Get your hormones, adrenals, and vitamin levels checked for deficiency or see if a supplement like melatonin helps.
8. Stay hydrated.
9. Try a sleep CD to help relax the mind and body.

All of these things will contribute to being better able to relax later and rest with peace for a healing sleep.

Food and Sleep Patterns

When you rest is when your body heals itself. I suggest you don't eat anything about three hours before bed. If your body has to digest and process food, then it's working. Allow it to rest and restore overnight, it needs to be free of chores and responsibilities. So give your body a break and have some soup for dinner or a light vegetarian meal. It would help to make your morning and lunch meal the main meals of the day.

If digestion is an issue, lie down on your left side for about 20 minutes.

According to Ayurveda healing tradition, when we sleep on the left side our lymphatic system drains more efficiently, it makes our heart beat easier, supports the spleen function, our bile flows easier and because of gravity, it encourages the food to move more effortlessly from the small intestine to the large intestine. "When you lie on the left side, the stomach and pancreas hang naturally, allowing for optimal and efficient digestion."[125]

Good advice comes from an old Ayurvedic remedy. If your body is acidic, try drinking a teaspoon of baking soda in a glass of water to neutralize the acid. What an easy, inexpensive solution! Drink healthy, hydrating fluids during the day, but don't drink too much right before bed. Then you won't have a need to get up in the middle of the night to go to the bathroom. Drinking herbal nighttime teas can also help promote rest and sleep.

Relaxing Bath

Consider taking an evening bath to relax and calm yourself before bedtime. Fill up a warm or hot bath and soak for ten minutes or more. I like to put mineral salts (Epsom salts or sea salt) in my bath. I also add organic apple cider vinegar to aid in adjusting my PH balance in my body. Then right before I step into the tub, I add a few drops of one of my favorite essential oils. I add it last so it won't evaporate before I can get in and enjoy the aroma. For nighttime and relaxation, my favorite is lavender oil.

My formula for my bath water is ¼ to ½ cup Epsom salts, ¼ cup of organic apple cider vinegar, and 5–10 drops of essential oil.

I have a water purifier on my showerhead and just fill my bath through my shower head. I don't like to have chlorine and fluoride in my shower and bath water because our skin absorbs things so quickly and easily. (That's why so many medicines are on patches.) Both chlorine and fluoride are carcinogens. Did you know that chlorine was the first chemical developed to kill in warfare? That's why I avoid it whenever I can. The purifier also removes fluoride and other toxins.

Peppermint, rosemary, and eucalyptus oils invigorate me, so I use those in the morning.

If you can't take a bath, a good foot soak can be beneficial and relaxing as well. When finishing a bath, make the final rinse a cool rinse to lock in the moisture to shrink the pores. After your shower or footbath, dry off and put on a soothing body lotion or cream to seal in the moisture. This helps avoid itchy, dry skin during the night.

If you're like me, you sleep better in comfortable clothing and sheets, so you might splurge on the quality of your bed linens and night clothes. It makes me feel better and I look forward to putting them on and getting into bed. I feel I'm pampering myself.

Air Purifier and Humidifier

I have an air decontamination (purifier) machine, which purifies the air in my home and in my bedroom. This machine cleans my air of mold, virus, fungus, and bacteria from the hard and soft surfaces as well as in the air. I also like the sound my portable machine makes, because it drowns out the sound of the outside world. There is an induct system that also works on the air conditioning system that makes no noise, if you prefer that. This air decontamination machine also makes the oxygen in my environment more bio available and easier to breathe. It is completely chemical free and can remove chemical contaminants from the environment safely and efficiently. I sleep so much more soundly, now that I am using this. This is an excellent machine for anyone who wants a healthier indoor environment or who has any kind of breathing problem. (See Resources.)

There are also humidifiers for winter when the heat can dry out the air. This can help with anyone who has trouble with nosebleeds in the winter. The inside of the nose gets too dry and can crack and cause bleeding. A cotton swab dipped in olive oil or coconut oil and rubbed inside the nostrils a few times a day will keep them moist and less likely to dry out and crack.

Doing this helped my family, especially when we were in high-altitude places in the winter.

Exercising and Hydrating

Getting exercise is another great way to sleep better at night. It can relieve stress and slow down your thinking. After all, you can't worry when you're moving and concentrating on what your body is doing. With exercise, oxygen circulates through your bloodstream, aiding digestion by moving your food through your system.

Exercise stimulates the body in many ways: by filling the lungs with fresher air, loosening muscles, getting your mind off the everyday patterns or worries, and helping to drain lymph glands. Be certain to hydrate when exercising. Drink a lot of good fluids, particularly hydrating fluids like fresh spring water, coconut water, water-rich vegetable or fruit juices, Rejuvelac, etc. The toxins in our body flushed out by exercise need to leave the body as quickly as possible. Drinking healthy hydrating fluids will help flush those toxins out of the body. Coconut water provides a natural electrolyte without the added sugar and chemicals of many processed sports drinks.

Deep Breathing and Massage

Along with exercise, engage in deep breathing, which is healing and relaxing. Breathe down deep in your diaphragm, taking long slow breaths as you finish exercising. Teach your children to breathe deeply. Getting oxygen moving though our bodies is highly valuable for our health. It overcomes a tendency to hold your breath, especially when you feel stressed. Not breathing cuts off the oxygen to the brain, which can stress you even more.

When you feel stressed, it helps to stop and consciously breathe deeply for three or more breaths. This will get oxygen to the brain and relax the whole body. If your mind won't stop, try counting when you breathe. For example, breathe in eight counts, hold for five counts, then exhale for eight counts. This takes your mind off "stuff" and provides a welcome break.

If you're unable to exercise, still be sure to breathe deeply, relax your mind, and do what you can to move. This helps drain your lymphatic system and keeps it clear from blockage. So does having a good massage periodically. In one yoga class I take, we do fast, deep breathing in and out of the nose for about three to five minutes. I can feel the oxygen pumping through my body and allowing my mind to release the subjects that keep popping into it.

Want a relaxing yoga pose that helps get the blood down to the head and heart from the feet? Put your bottom against a wall and your legs straight up the wall. Simply lie there on your back with the legs straight up and relax. This is an easy yoga exercise you can teach your children. I do this pose at every opportunity, especially if I've been on my feet all day or sitting all day when I'm traveling.

Because your organs are linked with nerves to your feet, when your feet hurt, your whole body can hurt. That's when it's wise to get a foot massage. You'll feel better and recover faster.

Create a Sacred Space

Make your bedroom a quiet, sacred place to sleep. Have all devices such as computer, TV, and cellphones out of the room, so they won't be emitting electromagnetic waves during your sleep. Don't have an electronic clock, radio, or alarm anywhere near your head. Place a device of this kind at least six feet away from your head or body.

Make your bedroom dark. Even the smallest light can disrupt sleep. Install blackout curtains or dark shades that can block out the light at any time. Don't have little nightlights, unless you really need them for safety. Use your own best judgment on this matter.

Have a peaceful break for about 20 or 30 minutes before going to sleep. Meditate on things that are positive, uplifting subjects. For example, write down things that you are grateful or thankful for, or read a positive, uplifting book or literature. What we have on our mind when we go to sleep can be crucial to what kind of sleep we have. Avoid news programs or violent shows, especially right before trying to get a good night's restful sleep. Whatever you have on your mind before going to sleep can be what can go over and over again in your mind for six to eight hours. So make sure it is something you want to have on your mind all night.

Affirmations

Every thought we have is an affirmation. Make every affirmation you have be something you want in your life. Don't think about problems; only think about solutions. Also think about what you *do* want in your life. What we concentrate on is what we can attract to our life, so make it the best things you can wish for. Be brave and concentrate on your heart's desire. Tell yourself that you go to sleep easily. What we tell ourselves has a huge impact on what actually happens to us. So remind the mind that it's time to rest.

Don't work in your bedroom or on your bed, if you can help it. Instead, make it a place where you rest and sleep. Set aside this space for calm meditation, relaxation, and peace. Make your bedroom a refuge from the outside world.

Remember, we're exposed to more information in 24 hours than our great grandparents were exposed to in a whole year. It is no wonder we get overloaded with too much information and too many responsibilities. So it is even more important to calm our minds and our space to get some positive rest and relaxation.

CHAPTER 18

Nontoxic Body Products and Therapeutic Hygiene

Body products are usually tested on animals or have ingredients in them that are toxic. This section contains some products that I have found to be better and/or made at home. You have many foods in your kitchen that are really easy, less expensive, and healthy to use in making your own beauty and bath products for your daily bathing routine. Making them yourself also ensures that you know exactly what is in your products. This is a fun activity to do with your children.

The skin is the largest organ of the body and readily absorbs the products you put on it. Products go straight to the blood vessels via patches, as mentioned earlier. The quality of ingredients is important. Buy organic if you have a choice.

Face Cleansers and Moisturizers

Honey is a natural moisturizer and has antibacterial properties. I use raw organic honey as my daily face cleanser. I love it because it makes my skin feel so smooth. Honey can also be used as a moisturizing mask. Put it on and leave for 10 or 15 minutes, and then remove it with a warm, wet washcloth. Your skin will feel moist and clean.

Extra virgin, pure organic coconut oil is extremely good for almost any skin but especially good for dry skin. I use it on my face and whole body.

Sesame seed oil pulls toxins from the skin. You can use it on your face or whole body. It has a little bit of a scent compared to coconut oil.

Face Masks

These are fun to make and do when you have daughters and slumber parties. My sisters and I used to make these when our friends came over. My daughter and I still do these together.

Avocado and cucumber mashed and blended together make a wonderfully refreshing, nutrient-dense mask. Cucumber slices can also be placed over the eyes to reduce swelling and redness.

Honey makes a very soothing and hydrating mask. Note: You can mix it with oatmeal and eggs for a nutrient-dense mask. Scrub it off with a warm, wet washcloth to exfoliate as well.

Yogurt is very calming and will help reduce redness of the skin. It makes a wonderful, cooling facial mask. Note: You can mix honey and/or eggs into yogurt, too. I like to experiment with ingredients. Strawberries and/or other fruits can be very nice to mash up and add. Experiment and find one that you love with the food you have on hand!

Eye Care

Warm, wet tea bags are great for reducing swollen, puffy eyes. The tannins in the tea work on the swelling. I use English breakfast or chamomile tea for this. I put a tea bag in a cup of warm water and let it sit for a moment.

I put an old, dark towel under my head (so my good towels don't get stained), and then I gently place a warm tea bag over each eye for about 15 minutes. It feels great and is so relaxing.

Exfoliating Skin

Combine almonds (ground into a meal) mixed with an equal amount of oatmeal, a little purified water or cucumber juice (enough liquid to make a nice paste), and some honey. Spread the mixture evenly on the skin and let dry. When it is dry, take a dry washcloth and rub the face to remove the mixture. This will exfoliate the dry, dead skin cells and clean out the pores. Then take a warm, wet washcloth, wash it off, and rinse well. Note: I use the almond meal I have left over from making my almond milk for this!

Body Scrubs, Moisturizers, Baths, and Foot Baths

Sea salt, a few drops of essential oil of your choosing, like eucalyptus or peppermint, and a little olive oil make a wonderful body scrub to remove dead skin and improve circulation. You can use sugar instead of sea salt, but since it goes right into your blood stream, I would use sea salt.

For a nice bath or foot soak, put mineral salts or sea salts in the bath with a little organic apple cider vinegar (to help adjust the pH balance of your body), and fill the tub with warm water. Right before you get in, add a few drops of eucalyptus oil and/or peppermint oil (to invigorate) or oil like lavender (to relax) to the bath or footbath. Put the oil in at the last minute or it will dissipate, and you won't get to really enjoy the aromatic effect.

You can add a few drops of your favorite essential oil to add a scent. (Note: I don't use the scented oil on my face, only on my body. I love using coconut oil.) I also like to put coconut oil mixed with peppermint or lavender oil on my feet and then put socks on for the night. These oils are refreshing. The socks help soften and nourish the dry skin on the feet.

Castor oil pulls toxins from the body. It is thick and gooey, but I have gotten used to it and use it fairly regularly on my face and body after showering. After I put it on my skin, I just put on my nice, thick robe and socks for a little while before I get dressed.

I have been using oils for my skin for many years. I had a beautician put purifying oils on me a few times, and I was hooked. I found that my skin felt so much better when I used natural oils instead of traditional lotions. Olive oil, pure coconut oil, jojoba oil, almond oil, and apricot oil all make wonderful body moisturizers/oils. Olive oil has a little fragrance.

My daughter puts olive oil all over her body in the shower just before getting out, and then quickly does her last rinse. She loves the way it makes her skin feel, and she doesn't have oil on her skin after she has dried off, even though her skin feels nourished, hydrated, and soft. Be careful not to slip in the shower if you do this, as olive oil can make the shower floor slippery.

Dry Skin Brushing

Skin brushing can do wonders for the whole body, mind, and spirit. I have done this for over 20 years and also did so for my children while raising them. Buy a natural bristle brush with a long handle, so you can reach body parts like the middle of your back. Wetting skin will not have the same effect. Try this for a week and see if you can get used to doing it.

Wonderful benefits from dry skin brushing include:

- Removing dead skin and cleaning out the pores of fresh skin.
- Tightening skin.
- Helping with digestion. (Since skin brushing stimulates the body muscles and the circulation system, it can also stimulate the body in continuing to move anything in the intestinal tract through the intestines.)
- Removing cellulite.
- Stimulating circulation.
- Increasing cell renewal.
- Strengthening the immune system.
- Stimulating and cleansing the lymphatic system and glands all over the body.

Try skin brushing every day before showering or bathing. Start with the feet. All ~~of~~ the body organs and nerve endings are connected to the feet, so when you treat the feet, you are also treating the whole body. You can work from the feet up the legs to the torso, and lastly the arms and hands.

- When brushing, always work upward in counter-clockwise circles toward the heart. It is all right to do this lightly where you are more sensitive. After you take a warm shower or bath, rinse with cool water to seal the skin and stimulate blood circulation. This will actually stimulate the surface warmth of the skin.
- Wash the skin brush every week in water and let it dry before using again.
- If you just can't do dry skin brushing, then try using a tough brush on your skin in the shower to really clean out the toxins and dirt from the pores. It will also help with circulation.

Hand Sanitizer/Hand Soap

Since antibiotic hand sanitizers have been on the market, many doctors believe they may be contributing to the development of super strains of viruses and bacteria. Also, they absorb right through our skin into our bloodstream, so using an antibacterial soap or hand sanitizer is basically like taking an antibiotic. The antibiotic kills all bacteria, including the good bacteria in our body that keep the bad bacteria in check. These good bacteria are a main part of our immune system. Before antibiotics were invented, natural oils and foods were used to help protect the body from pathogens.

In a *New York Times* article about Dr. Lawrence D. Rosen, a New Jersey pediatrician who makes and sells natural health advice and remedies, Rosen recommended his recipe for a homemade hand sanitizer called thieves oil.[126] His mixture of oils came from a legend about a group of 15th-century European perfumers who stole anything of value off dead bodies during the Bubonic Plague. They made a mixture of essential oils that had antibacterial and antiviral properties, and covered their bodies with the mixture. They also used this oil on their bodies to protect themselves from the germs—hence the name "thieves oil." Dr. Rosen's recipe includes equal amounts of therapeutic-grade essential oils: cinnamon bark, lemon, eucalyptus, clove, and rosemary. Mix the oils with coconut oil or jojoba oil as a carrier, and use it on hands as a sanitizer. For soap, you can mix it with a pure castile soap.

I use a mouthwash with this blend of oils in it as well. Essential oils are very potent. You may find it wise to do a skin test first, to make sure you don't have any adverse reactions to the oils of choice. In my opinion, these natural, antibacterial oil combinations are a great, natural alternative to the "antibiotic" versions.

Skin Care

One day when my children were small, I read about how the innocent Minnie Mouse Bubble Bath I'd just bathed my children in could cause blindness. I was so alarmed. So I started researching and reading ingredients on everything. How could the U.S. government allow toxin and carcinogenic ingredients in our toothpaste, bubble bath, shampoos, and more?

After going through my bathroom cabinets and reading all the ingredients, I threw out almost everything! Since then, I've been extremely careful about what I put on our bodies. Remember, what we put on our skin, our largest organ, is absorbed into the blood stream. Be sure to use safe, toxin-free products.

Look out for these ingredients:

- **DEA or Diethanolamine**. This ingredient is used in many household and personal products such as shampoo, bubble bath, lotions, and detergents for laundry or dishwashing. DEA is a known toxin in industrial applications, now proven to cause cancer when applied to the skin of rats. Dr. Samuel Epstein, author of *The Safe Shopper's Bible* and founder of The American Coalition to Prevent Cancer, is a leading authority on toxicology. He issued a strong warning about the use of cocamide DEA or lauramide DEA. Many products contain these ingredients and simply don't have warnings on them.[127]

- **Propylene Glycol.** This main ingredient in antifreeze and hydraulic fluids is used as a solvent. It's also found in pet food, lotions, shampoos, toothpastes, deodorants, processed foods, and more. A colorless, hygroscopic liquid, it has been tested by the American Academy of Dermatologists and found to cause skin irritation at low levels. It can be harmful if inhaled, ingested, or absorbed into the skin. It can also cause nausea, headaches, central nervous system depression, eye irritation, skin irritation, and gastrointestinal disturbances.
- **SLS or Sodium Lauryl Sulfate.** This is found in detergents, concrete cleaners, engine degreasers, and more. It's used in clinical studies to irritate skin tissue. It corrodes hair follicles and impairs the ability to grow hair. When combined with other nitrogen-bearing ingredients, carcinogenic nitrates can form. SLS enters (and maintains residual levels) in the heart, liver, lungs, and brain from skin contact.[128]
- **Talc.** Talcum powder is a mineral made up mainly of the elements silicon, magnesium, and oxygen. Talc is similar to asbestos and "may result in fallopian tube fibrosis with resultant infertility," according to the *Journal of the American Medical Association* (JAMA). "Talc's harmful effect on human tissue has been known for quite some time. Long ago, its dry lubricating properties were used as a glove-donning powder (easy to glide on) for surgical gloves. As early as the 1930s, talc was linked to post-operative granulomatous peritonitis and fibrous adhesions."[129]
- **Alcohol.** This is used in many mouthwashes. "Mouthwashes with a content of 25 percent or higher have been implicated in mouth, tongue, and throat cancers."[130]

Many people ask me what I put on my body and use for makeup. I use a certified organic make-up and skin care line by NYR Organic.

I love this English company's certified organic make-up, body care, baby products, essential oils, etc. People ask me what I wear. This is where I order my makeup, soaps, shampoos, essential oils, etc. I love the rose and frankincense products. The baby oil, shampoo, and similar products are terrific.

The mouthwash I use frequently and love is from Young Living, an essential oil company. A combination of antiviral, antibacterial essential oils is called Thieves. It's a blend of cinnamon, clove, lemon, eucalyptus, and rosemary.

As mentioned earlier, the Thieves name came from a band of spice traders who would cover themselves with oil and then rob dead people who had died of the Black Plague. They contributed never getting the plague to their use of these oils.[131] Note: Weber State University tested the oils and found it had a 99.96 kill rate with airborne bacteria.[132]

So, in conclusion, read ingredient labels and be savvy about protecting you and your family from toxic chemicals in your daily life.

Hair Care

Olive oil, coconut oil, argan oil, or mayonnaise can be used to moisturize and condition hair. Put it on the hair and place a plastic cap on it overnight (or even just for an hour or so), and then wash it out in the morning.

Letting your hair naturally dry as often as you can help your hair and scalp. Using a hair dryer is very drying and can cause brittle hair ends.

Nails and Cuticles

When you get out of the warm bath or shower and cuticles are soft and pliable, take your towel and gently push back each cuticle all the way around. This will keep cuticles receded and healthy, and you won't need to cut or trim them as much. You can also use a wooden cuticle stick to do this. Rub some oil into cuticles to keep them soft and from drying out. (I use any of the oils that I use after showering, like coconut, almond, olive, apricot, and castor oil.) Do this after a bath or shower; it can help seal in the moisture. Teaching children things like this is fun and easy.

Sore Throat and/or Stuffy Nose

For many years, my family went to Dr. Ludwig Michaels, an ear, nose, and throat doctor. He would clean our stuffy noses using a bulb syringe filled with a mixture of sea salt and warm water and gently pressed the mixture into each nostril. The water would come out the other nostril, along with any congestion. He repeated that process on each side a couple of times. We held our heads over a bowl to catch the water coming out. It always cleared up our congestion and was refreshing.

Neti pots work in the same way, but I don't think they are as easy to use as a bulb syringe. You can buy rubber bulb syringes and neti pots at many pharmacies.

Teeth, Gums, and Mouth Care

The mouth is highly absorbable. If you read the box of some name-brand toothpastes or mouthwashes, you may see a warning that if they are swallowed you should call poison control immediately. The warnings are usually only on the toothpaste box and not on the toothpaste tube itself. In my opinion, we shouldn't be putting any kind of poison in our mouths at all. I buy brands that are free of poison and not harmful to my body. I use an essential oil toothpaste and mouthwash.

Do not share your toothpaste. It can spread germs with others' toothbrushes brushing against the toothpaste opening.

Get a new toothbrush after any illness, or at least every two months. This will prevent the toothbrush from becoming too built up with germs. Use a tongue scraper to keep the tongue clean and fresh. Floss at least once daily to keep gums healthy and to remove bacteria from between teeth. Teaching children healthy hygiene habits is so beneficial for their long-term health.

Leslee's Fantastic Healing Deodorant

My dear friend Leslee Carr Feiwus makes the most wonderful, healthy deodorant for her family members. They love it and prefer not to use anything else.

Ingredients:

¼ cup arrowroot
¼ cup baking soda
¼ c. melted, organic coconut oil
20 drops of thieves oil for purification

Directions:

Combine all of the ingredients.
This recipe makes two small 2-ounce jars.

Note:

Leslee uses Young Living's antiviral, antibacterial essential oil called Thieves. You can use your own combination of antiviral, antibacterial essential oils. See resources.

CHAPTER 19

Natural Remedies

Growing up, I learned natural remedies from various people in my life. Many of these remedies have been passed down from generation to generation. Traditional natural remedies are a cherished and valued part of almost all cultures around the world. I have created a few remedies of my own based on my own research and with information from my doctors. What I like the most about these is that they are drug-free. This section contains some that I think are both easy and valuable.

The Magic of Chlorophyll

The amazing health benefits of using wheatgrass for healing were brought to the public's attention by Ann Wigmore in *The Wheatgrass Book: How to Grow and Use Wheatgrass to Maximize Your Health and Vitality.* When I started learning about cleansing, some 25 years ago, I started learning about the amazing positive effects grasses have on our body. I learned about barley grass as well as wheatgrass. The chlorophyll-rich grasses have enormous amounts of antioxidants and are highly alkalizing. There are many benefits of consuming juice freshly extracted from grasses. Here are some of the benefits, according to Ann Wigmore.[133] When externally applied to the skin, wheatgrass juice can:

- Help eliminate itching almost immediately.
- Soothe sunburned skin and act as a disinfectant.
- Soothe and heal cuts, burns, scrapes, rashes, poison ivy, athlete's foot, insect bites, boils, sores, open ulcers, tumors, and so on. (Use as a poultice and replace every two to four hours.)

When rubbed into the scalp before a shampoo, it can:

- Help mend damaged hair and alleviate itchy, scaly scalp conditions.
- Return gray hair to its natural color.

When the juice is gargled, it can:

- Sweeten the breath, and firm and tighten gums.

When the juice is consumed, it can:

- Greatly increase energy levels.
- Act as a beauty treatment that slows down the aging process.
- Cleanse your blood and help rejuvenate aging cells, slowing the aging process and making you feel more alive.
- Help tighten loose and sagging skin.
- Lessen the effects of radiation. (One enzyme found in wheatgrass, SOD, lessens the effects of radiation and acts as an anti-inflammatory compound that may prevent cellular damage following heart attacks or exposure to irritants.)
- Restore fertility and promote youthfulness.
- Work as a sleep aid. (Also place a tray of living wheatgrass near the head of your bed. It will enhance the oxygen in the air and generate healthful negative ions to help you sleep more soundly.)

Many health clinics in the United States today (including the Ann Wigmore Foundation and Retreat Center, Optimum Health Institute, Hippocrates Institute, and Tree of Life to name a few) use wheatgrass as a mainstay basic of their healing programs. The grass is high in antioxidants, oxygenates the blood, and is nutrient-dense. It is such an easy and simple healing modality.

Tea Tree Oil

When traveling with our children, I always took my tea tree oil and emergency food supply. Tea tree oil is antiseptic oil originally from Australia and New Zealand. The New Zealand type doesn't smell as strong as the other, yet it works really well. I order it through the mail because it's hard to find high-quality oils made in the U.S.

I used tea tree oil for almost everything once I learned what it did. Once when my son had chicken pox, I put full-strength tea tree oil on each spot. Miraculously, the spots were gone the next day. No itching, no scarring, no chicken pox. Why didn't everyone use this for chicken pox?

Here's when I was persuaded to look into this as an alternative cure. We were traveling in Greece and my son was bitten by something, perhaps a spider. He had a huge, red, painful, welt in the middle of his back. We had no clue how to find a doctor. It was late on a Sunday night. So I dabbed my tea tree oil on the spot a few times before he went to bed. And I prayed. He woke the next morning, and it was almost gone. How incredible. The swelling went away totally in a couple of days.

Another time, the contractor who was remodeling our house showed us his leg full of poison ivy. For more than a month, he'd gone to the doctor and tried everything—cortisone, creams, and more. When he put on my tea tree oil, his itching spots were remarkably better the next day. He kept putting it on and in less than a week, they had disappeared.

I love tea tree oil and I still use it for everything that looks like a welt or bite. My children now pack it when they travel. It is a good emergency treatment you can use for so many things.

The air gets very dry when we use heaters in our homes, particularly in the winter. A humidifier can really help. Adding a little eucalyptus or tea tree oil to the water in the humidifier adds a touch of natural antibacterial properties to the moist air. It also smells really good.

You can also use a cotton swab to coat the inside of the nostril with coconut oil or olive oil. This will moisten the skin lining the nostril and help it to not dry out and crack.

WATERMELON REMEDY FOR CONSTIPATION

Watermelon is one of the best remedies for constipation. It is packed with electrolytes and is very hydrating. Adding sea salt to this helps the body absorb more of the potassium in the watermelon.

Ingredients:

1 c. watermelon rind
1 c. watermelon
¼ tsp. unrefined, whole sea salt
1 c. string beans (optional)

Directions:

1. Wash the watermelon well.
2. Cut watermelon rind into bite-size pieces.
3. Juice about 1 to 2 cups of rind and a cup of the watermelon.
4. Juice the string beans as well, if using. This helps lower blood sugar. If the person is diabetic, add the strings beans in to be juiced with the watermelon.
5. Serve immediately.
6. Sprinkle lightly with whole sea salt.

◆ ◆ ◆

Honey and Cinnamon for a Variety of Ailments

The combination of honey and cinnamon has been used for centuries for many ailments. They both have powerful antibacterial properties. Canadian magazine *Weekly World News* listed the following diseases and conditions that can be cured by honey and cinnamon, according to research conducted by Western scientists: heart disease, insect bites, arthritis, hair loss, bladder infections, cholesterol, colds, infertility, upset stomach, gas, immune system issues, indigestion, pimples, skin infections, cancer, fatigue, bad breath, and hearing loss.[134]

Ceylon cinnamon is the best cinnamon to use. Cassia, Saigon, and Chinese cinnamon contain 5 percent coumarin, which can be problematic for the liver. Ceylon cinnamon has only .0004 percent coumarin.

HONEY-CINNAMON DRINK

Warning: Do not use honey with children under 18 months.

Ingredients:

1 T. honey, ¼ c. lukewarm water, 1 tsp. cinnamon

Directions:

Mix together all ingredients.

Note:

Drink on an empty stomach or before a meal.

◆ ◆ ◆

SLEEP AID

Warning: Do not use honey with children under 18 months.

Ingredients:

1 tsp. raw, unrefined honey

1 c. warm milk or chamomile tea

Directions:

1. Mix ingredients together.
2. Drink slowly.

SORE THROAT REMEDIES

1. Mix 1 tsp. honey (only for children over 18 months old) and 2 tsp. freshly squeezed lemon juice. Drink on an empty stomach, and then drink a glass of water 15–20 minutes later.
2. Gargle with warm sea salt and water.
3. Mash 1 garlic clove, let sit about 10 minutes, and then mix with some butter. Spread on a piece of bread or cracker and eat.

CHAPTER 20

A Walk Through the Grocery Store

Let me simply walk through the grocery store with you. Here are some ideas for going to the grocery store and what to look for.

Look for labels that say that the food is organic. You want organically grown and produced foods. The label may say "certified organic," meaning that it had the certification issued from the USDA. If it is organic, it was supposed to be grown from seed that was not genetically engineered. (I do see canola oil that is certified organic, and it is a genetically engineered seed. Alas, this is a discrepancy, because the USDA says it doesn't allow genetically engineered seeds to be used.) There are two basic types of genetically engineered crops on the market now: herbicide-tolerant and insect-resistant.

Herbicide-tolerant crops usually include corn, cotton, sugar beets, soy, and canola. These are grown to handle the direct use of pesticides on them. There are over a billion pounds of pesticides used in the United States alone each year. Many of these chemical fertilizers were developed for use as bombs or poisons in warfare. They poison our food and our environment. Pesticides particularly affect our nervous system.

These chemicals can also destroy the sulfur in the soil. Food grown in that way does not contain sulfur, which helps our bodies absorb oxygen into our cells. It's another reason to eat food grown without chemicals.

Insect-resistant crops usually include corn, potatoes, soy, and cotton. These plants actually produce an insecticide to kill insects that feed on them or have a toxin built into them. An example is the Bt toxin that is supposed to only eat holes in the stomachs of the insects to kill them. Studies are now showing that they are actually eating holes in the people that ingest these foods as well. I would avoid these foods completely.

Watch out for corn and soy, used as fillers in many processed foods. I'm assuming most of the corn and soy is genetically modified. This harmful corn and soy can also enter our bodies through meat from animals that have ingested them. In my opinion, we really need to have a federal law requiring genetically modified foods (GMO) be on food labels. The effect of this type of plant on the environment and in the human body, especially long term, is unknown.

Genetically engineered or genetically modified (GM) plants are escaping into the wild and interbreeding with wild plants. Our pollinators, such as bees, are in trouble now. Are genetically engineered plants a contributing factor? Good question. Genetically engineered food is such a recent phenomenon that no in-depth studies show their long-term effect on humans or the ecosystem. You must decide for yourself if eating food that has pest control built right into it or has large amounts of poisons put on it is good for human consumption.

According to an article on Dr. Joseph Mercola's website, "An estimated 75 percent of foods in U.S. grocery stores contain GM ingredients. About seven out of every 10 items in the average grocery cart have been genetically modified. And don't bother reading labels to see if you're buying a GM product, because at this time *no labeling is required.*"[135]

Organic food is supposed to be grown without chemical, synthetic, or biological pest control or fertilizers. Although the USDA continues to water down its regulations, certified organic is still better than noncertified organic. This is because the USDA organic label gives you the most information about the origins and production of your food. These foods must adhere to much stricter regulations than any other food on the market, and the stricter the regulations, the more you will know about what is actually in your food, thus giving you more control over what you put into your body and empowering you to make more informed decisions at the grocery store.

You may want to let your voice be heard in favor of stricter food labeling and production regulations. Personally, I would like to see foods containing genetically modified ingredients labeled as such, as is currently required in most Western countries. If you would like to make your voice heard, call your local representatives and senators and let them know how you feel. Join the Organic Consumers Association (www.organicconsumers.org) and keep up with the bills and laws.

Produce

Start by trying to buy fruits and vegetables that are in season. They will be fresher and less expensive. Most fruits and vegetables in our stores are about five days old. They are harvested, packed, shipped, and unpacked before we buy them.

When food is harvested, it continues to have living enzymes, which fade and die as time passes. Therefore, the more recently the food is harvested, the more enzymes it contains.

I suggest you carefully examine the food you buy. Select undamaged produce that smells fresh and has smooth, firm skin. Also, look for vibrancy of color. The antioxidants are in the color pigment; therefore, the more color, the higher the antioxidant content. Avoid buying produce with bruises, cuts, or mold. If it's in a plastic bag or container, inspect it with extra care. Try to buy organic produce thatisn't artificially colored, waxed, or dipped to make it look commercially better for market.

Our body needs food that is in season because it works in harmony with the earth. Food grown locally is fresher, more flavorful, and usually more cost effective. The freshest food is ripened "on the vine" and then picked and eaten as soon as possible.

As I mentioned, I highly recommend always buying certified organic food. Support the farmers who are not poisoning the environment, and buy food that is free of pesticides and chemical fertilizers. Children are much more sensitive to these poisons because their organs are still forming.

All pesticides are not created equal. Some are worse than others. The following may help you decide what you should buy nonorganic.

Foods with the highest use of pesticides:

- Apples
- Bell Peppers
- Celery
- Cherries
- Grapes
- Lettuce
- Nectarines
- Peaches
- Pears
- Potatoes
- Spinach
- Strawberries
- Cherry tomatoes
- Snap peas (imported)
- Kale/collard greens
- Hot peppers

Foods that usually have the lowest use of pesticides:

- Avocados
- Asparagus
- Bananas
- Broccoli
- Cabbage
- Corn
- Kiwi
- Mangoes
- Onions
- Papaya
- Pineapples
- Eggplant
- Grapefruit

- Cantaloupe
- Cauliflower
- Sweet Potatoes

Clean all fruits and vegetables before you eat them. Apple cider vinegar works well and isn't very expensive. Use 1 tablespoon for each gallon of water, or ¼ cup for a sink full of water. Let fruits and vegetables soak at least 15 minutes. I clean everything, even things I peel (like avocados) because the knife that cuts through food will pull toxins from the outer skin into the food.

Mushrooms

When the weather is cold, I love something savory and hearty like mushrooms, which are surprisingly rich in nutrients. These dense, smooth, earthy fungi grow in thousands of varieties and have been studied extensively for their health benefits. Studies show that mushrooms aid the immune system because they are rich in antioxidants, potassium, selenium, copper, riboflavin, niacin, and pantothenic acid. In addition, select mushrooms are one of only two natural food sources of vitamin D. One medium Portobello mushroom has 407 mg of potassium, compared to a small banana at 362 mg, while an orange has 237 mg and four or five small button mushrooms have 237 mg. Selenium is an important mineral that works as an antioxidant to protect the body and support the immune system. Four or five medium crimini mushrooms have 21.8 mcg of selenium, as compared to one large egg with 15 mcg, or three ounces of lean beef with 18.1 mcg, a portobello mushroom with 9.2 mcg, or four or five white mushrooms with 7.8 mcg. In addition, the copper in mushrooms helps make red blood cells, which carry oxygen throughout the body.

When you buy them, look for mushrooms that are smooth, clean, and fresh in appearance. Keep them in the same container they come in, and refrigerate them until you're ready to use them. To clean them, use a soft mushroom brush or wet paper towel to remove any parts that look dirty or mushy. You can rinse them, but do not soak them. They can keep up to a week in the refrigerator in a porous paper bag, but never put mushrooms in an airtight container and never freeze them. Also, always trim the end of the stem before you use mushrooms. Many of the stems are too tough, so just use the caps if this is the situation.

There is a huge variety of mushrooms, thousands of which are poisonous, so do *not* pick them in the wild. Always buy them from a reliable and reputable supplier.

Adding mushrooms to dishes is easy. Thinly slice some mushrooms and put them on salads, in pasta dishes, or on sandwiches, or serve them as a side dish. Grilling them is always great, and mushrooms make a good vegetarian alternative to a burger. I love to sauté them with onions and butter to bring out the rich flavor of savory mushrooms. Each mushroom has a different flavor, so experiment and try a different variety every now and then.

Sprouts

Why does this food have its own section? Because sprouts are so incredibly nutritious and power-packed, they simply need their own section!

Sprouts are the ultimate superfood, the basis of life. They rejuvenate, reenergize, and heal. Sprouts are one of the most complete and nutritionally rich sources of all foods tested for nutrients. Sprouts can contain all the nutritional value of the whole plant in one little sprout!

The Chinese have included sprouts as a nutritional part of their diet for thousands of years. The mung bean is one of my favorite sprouts. A sprouted mung bean has the carbohydrate content of a melon, vitamin A of a lemon, thiamin of an avocado, riboflavin of a dry apple, niacin of a banana, and ascorbic acid of a loganberry—in one sprout!

In a newspaper article by Linden Staciokas, Dr. Paul Talalay of the American Cancer Society is quoted as saying that "broccoli sprouts are better for you than full-grown broccoli, and contain more of the enzyme sulforaphane which helps protect cells and prevents their genes from turning into cancer."[136]

Sprouts are a complete food containing protein, carbohydrates, and "good" fat. They are rich in vitamins, minerals, and natural enzymes. Studies have shown that when seeds and grains are germinated, they increase in nutrients and enzymes "25 to 4,000 percent."[137] Because of the protein shortage during World War II, Dr. Clive M. McKay promoted sprouted soybeans as a wartime food source.

Add sprouts to salads, sandwiches, dips, smoothies, green drinks, juices, and more!

Bulk Foods

Some fruits come in packages of four or more. Buying these packages is often more cost-effective than buying them separately. Be sure to check fruit for bruises, cuts, and freshness.

Nuts, seeds, grains, rice, soup mixes, granola, trail mixes, and more can be found in the bulk foods section. These can be less expensive, and there may be more turnover in this area of the store, so the food is often fresher than what is already bagged or packaged. Be certain to read the ingredients completely to see if they have added sugar or any other ingredients you are not expecting, and make sure they have an organic label. Nut butters, maple syrup, honey, and purified water are usually in this section at Whole Foods Market.

Spices, herbs, and tea are great items to buy in bulk. There is a greater turnover in these items as well, and they will probably be fresher than the prepackaged varieties. Also, you can get the exact amount you need for a dish rather than being left with an entire bottle of a spice or herb you don't use often.

Buying bulk spices, herbs, teas, and salts whole and grinding them yourself, or buying them ground in small amounts as needed, is a good practice and likely gives you a fresher product. Store fresh spices, herbs, and teas in airtight glass containers so they keep longer and stay fresher.

Read the Ingredients

Know what is in the food and body products that you buy. The front label of a product can be very misleading. I learned a long time ago that "natural" means nothing. Foods can be completely chemically derived and still say "natural" on the advertisement or package. The U.S. Code of Federal Regulations says a natural flavor or flavoring is: "the essential oil, oleoresin, essence or extractive, protein hydrolysate, distillate, or any product of roasting, heating or enzymolysis, which contains the flavoring constituents derived from a spice, fruit or fruit juice, vegetable or vegetable juice, edible yeast, herb, bark, bud, root, leaf or similar plant material, meat, seafood, poultry, eggs, dairy products, or fermentation products thereof, whose significant function in food is flavoring rather than nutritional.'[138]

In the book *Fast Food Nation*, Eric Schlosser wrote that consumers prefer to see the words "natural flavors' on a label, believing they are healthier. But the distinction between artificial and natural flavors can be arbitrary and somewhat absurd, based more on how the flavor has been made than on what it actually contains.[139]

He also wrote that a natural flavor is not necessarily healthier or purer than an artificial one. When almond flavor (benzaldehyde) is derived from natural sources, such as peach and apricot pits, it contains traces of hydrogen cyanide, a deadly poison.[140]

A product may say olive oil is in the product, but the ingredients may list canola oil or something else as well, or a larger amount than what was advertised on the packaging. Shop prepared: Take your reading glasses with you, because ingredients are printed so small sometimes that they can be very difficult to read. Foods like bread, crackers, and pasta can also be very misleading. Read ingredient lists carefully. Look for chemicals and additives.

Take pasta, for example. Pasta is a product that should be purchased as a whole grain. Read the label and make certain that it says "whole grain" and that it has the same ingredients that the packaging indicates it has. There are good whole-grain pastas, some of which are even gluten-free, like spelt, rice, and quinoa (which is really a seed) pasta. Quinoa is also a complete protein, so it is a good choice for vegetarians or vegans. Sprouted grains are also more digestible, so look for any kind of sprouted grains in breads, crackers, cereals, etc.

Raw food sometimes contains a great deal of sugar, so always check the amount. I try not to buy foods with agave nectar, corn or rice syrup, canola oil, or non-whole-grain flour. And remember that "natural" means nothing in labeling. Companies also use the term "natural" as an alias for adding MSG to food. Be aware of this and look for natural flavorings, coloring, and so forth on ingredient lists. If in doubt, ask a store employee for more information about a product. Shop at a store where employees go out of their way to help with any questions or concerns you may have about their products.

Read labels carefully. Products marked "low-fat" or "fat-free" are usually less healthy than the full-fat versions. This is just a marketing gimmick. Many of these products have added sugar or white refined salt, and may actually have chemicals in them.

Beware of the power of advertising; it can lead you to believe you are buying one thing when you are really being sold something else. Packaging is big business, and it can be misleading. Be a smart and savvy shopper.

Packaging

Most cans are lined with BPA, which is a synthetic estrogen and hormone disruptor. I asked a Whole Foods market employee about their brand products, and he told me they don't use the BPA to line their cans. I also see other companies putting BPA-free on the label.

BPA-free packaging can be found. Look for BPA-free packaging or the numbers on plastic packaging, which will indicate if it is safe. Safer plastic packages will be numbered 1, 2, 4, 5, and 6. When all is said and done, however, glass is always the safest option.

Baking Section

In many stores, this section has extra-virgin olive oil, extra- virgin, pure coconut oil, ghee, apple cider vinegar, unrefined sea salt, spices, yeast, various types of flours and sugars, other oils, parchment paper and baking needs.

Asian Foods

This area of the store should contain different types of soy sauces, miso, plum paste, and seaweed varieties. Freeze-dried soups and foods are good to pack for travel emergency meals, emergency meals for home, or camping. These don't usually require a can opener and can be used in many situations with only a little water added to hydrate them.

Snack Food Bars, Chocolate Bars, Protein Bars, and Raw Food Bars

Read labels. Make sure what is advertised is what is listed in the ingredients! Whey is a dairy. I do not recommend this as a food bar ingredient. Many good food bars that are raw, organic, and made with whole foods and/or protein (made up of sprouted grains, nuts, seeds, and other ingredients) do not contain whey or soy. Check the sugar and salt content. Many contain agave nectar, which can have an even higher glycemic index than high-fructose corn syrup. Be aware of this if you have high blood sugar.

Coconut water is usually on the shelves in this area with the health food bars or "raw" food bars. Coconut water is rich in electrolytes. It was used in many wars as a substitute for blood when blood was needed but unavailable for blood transfusions. Coconut water shares many of the same properties as human blood. It is extremely hydrating and rich in nutrients. It is a great post-workout drink or water alternative.

Superfoods and/or Raw Foods

Superfoods are foods that have more nutrients in them than many "normal" everyday foods.

These foods are usually grown in rainforests or areas where the soil is still rich in nutrients. Raw, vegan, gluten-free superfoods are usually in an area all by themselves. You can find meal-replacement protein powder that is raw, vegan, organic, and gluten-free, green concentrated powders, chia seeds, cacao powder, goji berries (wolf berries), acai berries, golden berries, and maca root.

Frozen Foods

Stores usually offer many choices of breads, imitation meats, easy meals, healthy ice creams, and frozen fruits and vegetables. Most growers who freeze their produce do so within hours of the produce being picked, so frozen foods may be more nutrient-dense than some fresh foods. Frozen fruits are good in smoothies, and they make smoothies colder without getting watery from adding ice. Some raw food practitioners think that freezing food changes it molecularly. Many raw food people don't eat or buy frozen foods. Decide what works for you, and live your life accordingly.

Breads, Crackers, and Chips

Have you ever been in the bread or cracker aisle at the supermarket, with all the choices of "all natural," "whole wheat," "whole grain," "sprouted," and "organic"? These are some words that have become really attractive to us, especially if we are trying to buy the healthiest foods. However, these words on food packaging can be misleading.

By labeling standards, products are required to use only a small percentage of whole-grain ingredients in order to list "whole grain" on their label. A product can be mostly white, refined flour and still have "whole grain" or "whole wheat" on the label, as long as there's some whole grain or whole wheat in it. Look to see that "100% whole organic grain" or "100% whole wheat" is the very first ingredient listed, so you are not tricked into buying a product made of mostly white, refined wheat, or other flour that has had the nutrition-rich part of the grain removed.

Ingredients are listed in order of the amount used in the product. Most of the nutrients are in the germ of the grain, and the hull is the fiber. When these are removed (as is the case with white flour), the grain is left devoid of nutrients or fiber, and the body uses it as if it were sugar.

The first four to five ingredients are especially important because they make up the bulk of a product. Wheat has a unique ability to raise blood sugar extremely quickly.

Blue corn has 20 percent more protein, 8 percent less starch, and a lower glycemic index than yellow corn. If you are buying chips or tortillas, look for the blue kind.

You'll find a variety of chips made with bean flour or other types of grain or seed flour. Buy multigrain or bean flour chips that are organic and have low sugar content.

"Sprouted" is another term seen in food products today. When a grain is sprouted, it makes the grain much more digestible. Many bread, cracker, and cereal products today have sprouted grains listed on the package or in the ingredient list. Look for the words "sprouted whole grain" in the list of ingredients.

Our thyroid is our master gland. It is central to all of our body's major functions. It influences our metabolism, digestion, energy, body temperature, skin, hair, sleep, mental acuity, nervous system, sexual organs, and hormonal system. In fact, it would be very difficult to find a system that is *not* influenced by the thyroid. The main nutrient that supports our thyroid is iodine. Up until 1980, bakeries added iodine to bread. After that they switched to potassium bromate.

What does this mean? We have a certain amount of space for the iodine in our thyroid. When we ingest potassium bromate, it acts like iodine. It will take up the space for iodine and actually prevent your body from absorbing the iodine it needs. This contributes to iodine deficiency. Check ingredient lists or ask at the bakery if potassium bromate is put in the bakery goods.

According to the Center for Science and Public Interest (CSPI), the FDA has known that bromate causes cancers in laboratory animals, but has failed to ban it. Canada banned it in 1994 and Great Britain in 1990.[141] "The FDA should fulfill its responsibility to protect the public's health," said Michael F. Jacobson, PhD, executive director of CSPI.[142] Instead of meeting privately with the potassium bromate industry, the FDA should ban bromate immediately. When the FDA tested foods in 1992–1993 and again in 1998–1999, many baked goods contained unsafe levels of potassium bromate.

Check packages of Pepperidge Farm, Pillsbury, and Best Foods, Inc. (maker of Arnold, Entenmann's, and Oroweat products.) They say they have switched to bromate-free processes. Make sure you read the ingredient list of bakery goods for this ingredient.

Grains

Buy organic sprouted grains, rice, and beans in the freshest, most whole form that you can. The nutrients are in the germ, right below the hull. The hull is the fiber, and the germ is the nutritious part. So, for the most nutritious food, buy whole grains in all of the choices of grains and rice. This is one of the best ways to get protein. Grains are inexpensive and delicious, and there is a huge variety. When ready to use, rinse grains well. Grains have been milled and stored in storage units or silos (probably in a place where bugs, mice, rats, and snakes can be found). I use a fine, mesh colander to rinse grains.

Organic, Local Milk, Cheese, and Eggs

One weekend I visited local organic farms just outside of Dallas. I wanted to see for myself if what I had been told at the farmer's market was really true. I was so amazed at the information I learned on this adventure. Some of these farms are completely organic, but not certified. It costs another five or six thousand dollars to get certified, and some farmers don't produce enough to make it worth their effort and money to become organically certified. Other farms I visited did have the certification.

Some farms I visited raised goats (for fresh, raw goat milk), chickens (for eggs), and/or cows for dairy. These farms were impressive. They were incredibly healthy and well managed. Some of them pumped water from their clean pond (never used by the animals for bathing) to the animals' drinking troughs. All of the animals were out in a large green pastures with shade trees and room to roam and play.

These farmers taught me a lot about certain types of labeling. Farmers use many different labels on packages of eggs, poultry, and milk products. Chickens in large farming practices can be called "free-range" if they have access to a place where they can move around, even if it's a cement room that they never even get to go into. Chickens can be called cage-free if they are not in cages. "Cage-free" can mean a huge, overcrowded room of chickens that can barely move. "Free-roaming" means they have 18 inches of dirt; it does not mean grass, fresh air, or sunlight. Look for eggs in cartons labeled "pasture raised" humanely with a certain amount of feet per chicken.

The cows at the farm I visited are 100 percent grass fed. I learned that more antacids are used on cattle in feedlots and factory farms than on humans. Cows that eat what I call "not normal" food ("normal" being grasses and green vegetation from the land) have trouble digesting grains and seed oils and can have terrible stomach acid. Animals that are fed organic food aren't necessarily fed the natural food these animals would normally eat in the wild. They can be organically raised but not be eating properly for their species. Stress breaks down the immune system, so stressed animals will have a weakened immune system. Also, if the cow is fed corn that is genetically modified with Bt toxin, that Bt toxin can be passed into your system as well. The Bt toxin can create holes in the stomach or intestinal tract. Therefore, I recommend buying beef or animal meat raised on organic grass or has been fed an organic, natural diet.

The owner of the farm I visited moves animals from pasture to pasture without rough cowboys. In fact, it is done in a calm and loving way that allows the land to "rest" and acquire the nutrients from manure the animals leave on the pastures. Each pasture is allowed to rest two to four months before putting the animals back. This way, the grasses to grow back after taking in the nutrients of the composted manure. The soil was very healthy, as seen by the worm castings everywhere I walked. (Worms thrive in healthy soil.)

Grass-fed cows can be fed grain and are often fed grain and/or seed oil (such as cotton seed oil) to fatten them. Animals suffer and consequently so do consumers because of these practices.

For the best milk and cheeses, find a 100 percent grass-fed herd and an operation that does not pasteurized its milk and cheese. This means it has the live enzymes and probiotics in a greater quantity than in the pasteurized versions. As mentioned earlier, milk and cheese from goats are more digestible for humans than cow milk.

Most cities have farms in the area that grow food and raise animals in an organically sound way. Find groups that support organic, fresh, slow foods and see if there is a co-op for organic food in the area. Also go to meet-ups or co-ops online in your area and find a group. (Check out www.localharvest.org.)

The next time you are in the supermarket and see cheaply priced eggs, milk, and cheese, think about why they are so cheap. When you buy from a small farmer with organic, healthy, environmentally friendly farming practices, you are voting with your pocketbook for these farmers to survive and thrive.

When making food choice transitions, many of us may need to take baby steps toward new food choices. Vegan and alternative milks and cheeses are delicious, but they do taste a little different. Try tasting them first and adding them to your diet a little at a time. I added nondairy milks to my milk a little each time I had it before I eventually switched.

Vegan, raw-food nut cheeses are delicious. Let your taste buds start to change in that direction. We develop new taste buds on a continual basis. If you want to "learn" to like something, start eating it regularly (at least 10 times or for two weeks). You will find that your taste buds will adjust.

Dairy is hard for many people to digest. When mammals are born, they have a lactase enzyme to help digest their mother's milk. By about age four, mammals lose most of that enzyme, so digesting milk is much harder. Also, milk products that are pasteurized are acidic in nature, and our pH balance is very important to maintain health. The dairy industry advertises calcium in milk, but if it is acidic, our body can pull calcium from the bones in order to adjust the pH balance from all the acidic dairy being consumed.[143]

If you are worried about iron, dairy is not a good thing to consume. A study reported in the *American Journal of Clinical Nutrition* in 1987 said that the calcium from dairy products impairs absorption of iron and blocks its transport across the cells lining in the small intestines.[144] In the book *Fit For Life II,* Harvey and Marilyn Diamond say, "Dairy products are disease producing."[145]

Think about finding alternatives to dairy in your diet. I put one of my clients on a dairy-free diet, although she didn't think she could do it. Within one week, she said she had no more acid reflux disease and was sleeping all night for the first time in a long time. In addition to trying goat milk, I recommend using organic, raw, unpasteurized milk products from a reliable organic source—a facility and animals in extremely healthful environments with fresh air, sunshine, exercise, and healthy, natural food. You'll find good raw cheese vegan cheese recipes in Alissa Cohen's living food books (Living *on Live Food* and *Raw Food for Everyone)* as well as in this book

Cheese and Jelled Food

When I first became vegetarian, I didn't realize animals' stomach substances are put in cheese to make it firm. It is called rennet. This is a meat product. This may not bother you, but I don't want to eat that. So I now look for cheese that has "vegetable enzymes" instead.

Gelatin capsules are also meat-based. Gelatin is taken from the hooves or nails and hair of animals. Look for vegetarian capsules made with things like agar. Agar is a seaweed extract that can be used instead of gelatin, and you can substitute it for gelatin in recipes most of the time. It does need to be heated in order to dissolve. Rather, it needs to be dissolved slowly and with continual stirring.

When making a Jell-O type of fruit dish, use agar flakes. Heat them slowly while stirring constantly. The flakes will dissolve from the middle toward the outside of the mixture. Combine this dissolved agar flakes mixture with fruit juices for a nice jelled dish.

CHAPTER 21

Buying Basic Kitchen Equipment

Once you've made a commitment to eat better, what equipment do you buy to support that commitment? Here are my suggestions:

1. Blender. A blender is probably my most useful kitchen tool. I use it almost every day. Vitamix is a good brand and has a seven-year warranty, but it costs more than most blenders. I am hard on my blenders and would wear out a blender about every three months. Then I bought my Vitamix. I love it. Mine is 15 years old now and still working great. Breville and the KTec Champ HP3 blenders are both good as well. With a normal blender, soak hard foods in water overnight to soften them so they won't be so hard on your blender.
2. Juicer. The Breville juicer is fairly easy to use and reliable. I juice carrots and a cucumber almost every day. You cannot juice wheatgrass or sprouts in this type of blender. I tried the Green Star brand, but it wore out fairly quickly with a good deal of use with large vegetables. The Hurom juicer does the same thing as the Green Star. One of my friends has the Hurom juicer and says it works great. She loves it.
3. Food processor. Food processors are very useful for making large amounts of raw food or mixing dense or heavy foods, like hummus. Small ones work just fine for most jobs. They have really small food processors for making small amounts, like baby food. If I were buying a large one, I would only buy a 10-inch one. My 12-inch has a gap that, in my opinion, doesn't

work as well.

4. Stainless steel rice cooker. The Lotus brand has become one of my absolute favorite appliances. It cooks rice, quinoa, and lentils perfectly, and then keeps them warm until it's time to serve. Lotus Foods Rice Cooker and Vegetable Steamer has an inner cooking pot and steaming tray that are constructed completely of mirror-finish stainless steel. I loved it so much, I gave both my daughter and son one of them.
5. Toaster/toaster oven. Choose one of good quality.
6. Paring knife and/or large cutting knife. Choose high quality.
7. Cutting board. If you have a dishwasher, buy a cutting board that is dishwasher-safe so that it can be sanitized completely.
8. Stainless steel sieve.
9. Spatula and scraper.
10. Glass, stainless steel, or lead-free ceramic baking dishes.
    Note: Be careful about Pyrex dishes. A Chinese company that bought the company changed the formula, and now some of the glass cookware has been exploding in heated ovens.[146] I look for old Pyrex dishes at antique stores and estate sales. Aluminum cookware can leach aluminum into the food. (Aluminum is linked to Alzheimer's disease.[147])

Note:

Avoid nonstick cookware. Studies show it releases toxins into the air when heated to high temperatures. "There's a whole chemistry set of compounds that will come off when Teflon is heated high enough to decompose," says Robert L.Wolke, PhD, a professor emeritus of chemistry at the University of Pittsburgh. "Many of these are fluorine-containing compounds, which as a class are generally toxic."[148] Explains Kurunthachalam Kannan, PhD, an environmental toxicologist at the New York State Department of Health's Wadsworth Center, "At temperatures above 500° F, the breakdown begins and smaller chemical fragments are released."[149] People don't want those toxins in their systems.

Using a Microwave

Yes, life is all about energy. Our food contains a certain type of energy, yet that every gets changed when food is microwaved.

Microwaving your food bombards the food with chaotic energy, distorting the molecular structure and destroying the nutrients. My former husband, an environmental trial lawyer, studied microwave ovens when they were first introduced to the market. Since then, he has never allowed a microwave in his home.

A study conducted and presented by the Department of Pediatrics at Stanford University School of Medicine noted this: "Microwaving appears to be contraindicated at high temperatures, and questions regarding its safety exist even at low temperatures."[150]

Even with this said, we consume our food for its nutrient value. "Broccoli is prized as a healthy food in part because it contains high levels of chemicals believed to protect against heart disease and some kinds of cancer. Now a new study from Spain suggests that health lovers hoping to get those benefits keep their broccoli away from the microwave. The study, published in the November issue of the *Journal of the Science of Food and Agriculture* found that broccoli cooked by microwave lost 74 percent to 97 percent of its antioxidant compounds, which are believed to be healthful. The researchers from the University of Murcia at Espinardo found by contrast that broccoli cooked by steaming lost less than 10 percent of the same chemicals."[151,152]

Microwaves directly affect the cell structure and water molecules in food. Knowing how vital the quality of water is for our body, I will never knowingly use or consume food from a microwave oven.

CHAPTER 22

How to Stock Your Pantry in a Healthy Way

What basic things are needed to have in a well-stocked, healthy kitchen? Here is a list of my pantry basics.

Foods to Keep on Hand

SEA SALT

Use solar-dried or mined, organic sea salt. This is essential for its minerals. Good-quality, unrefined salt will have about 65 trace minerals. Sea salt is good for you, and will make the flavor of your food more vibrant and tasteful. Salt is very grounding and can strengthen different parts of the body. It has an alkalizing effect on the body. Natural sea salt is not the same as the processed, bleached brands of salt. It won't have iodine in it, so take an iodine supplement unless you eat a great deal of seaweed.

SWEETENERS

Xylitol is a little grainier than white refined sugar, but look at the benefits of using it! Xylitol has antimicrobial effects of preventing the growth of bacteria. Xylitol is also alkaline enhancing and can replace sugar in recipes in equal substitution. It tastes and looks just like sugar with no bitter aftertaste. Xylitol has been shown to help prevent cavities, repair dental enamel, regulate blood sugar for those with type 2 diabetes, strengthen bones, decrease age-related bone loss, inhibit serious systematic yeast problems, inhibit the growth of bacteria that cause middle-ear infections in young children, inhibit the growth of streptococcus pneumonia, and alleviate dry mouth. Xylitol has 40 percent fewer calories and 75 percent fewer carbohydrates than sugar. Xylitol is slowly absorbed and metabolized, which results in negligible changes in insulin. Studies have shown that consumption of xylitol can reduce sugar cravings, reduce insulin levels, and alkalize your body.

Stevia: This is a sweet plant that has no calories. I like the liquid ones best. You just need a drop or two in place of each teaspoon of sugar. Stevia is a good choice for diabetics and/or anyone who wants a healthy, sweet flavor. The Sweet Leaf brand comes in flavors (vanilla, toffee, orange, etc.). I use it to sweeten my tea, nut milks, smoothies, and more.

Honey: Natural, raw honey has antibacterial and antitoxic properties. It has been used for centuries for burns, sore throats, and stomach disorders. Most honey on the market today is not raw. Make sure you are buying unprocessed, raw and local honey. Note: Never give honey to a child under 18 months old.

Maple syrup: This is boiled down from maple tree sap, and is light and sweet.

BLACK PEPPER

Buy whole, raw peppercorns and use a pepper grinder.

VINEGAR

Buy raw, unrefined vinegar. (In order for the body to process distilled vinegar, it causes the body to pull minerals from the body, so, I don't recommend buying distilled vinegar to be used in the making of food.) I really like raw, unrefined, organic apple cider vinegar. It is antiparasitic, is antifungal, neutralizes poisons, helps with blood circulation, and more. Balsamic vinegar is great to keep in the pantry for making salad dressings or as a dip or spread to use with bread.

I use vinegar for cleaning my fruits and vegetables, before cooking or juicing, by soaking them in water mixed with unrefined apple cider vinegar.

TEA

The best teas, in my opinion, are unprocessed and organic. Tea can be used for calming and refreshing the body. Tea can also be used medicinally and ceremoniously.

SPICES

I use Ceylon cinnamon, thyme, parsley, and turmeric frequently. Buy spices in small quantities so that you know they are fresh.

COCONUT OIL

Raw, unprocessed, organic, extra-virgin, pure coconut oil is a great choice for all recipes that call for oil.

EXTRA-VIRGIN OLIVE OIL

Buy organic, extra-virgin olive oil in dark glass bottles. Keep this refrigerated.

HIGH-QUALITY WATER

I always keep clean, pure, structured water (free of chlorine and fluoride), in my kitchen. It's used for all of my cooking or food preparation needs.

CHAPTER 23

Nontoxic Household Cleaning Products

All of these products you'll find in this chapter are safe, nontoxic, and not tested on animals. Most can even save you money.

BORAX POWDER

Twenty Mule Team Borax Natural Laundry Booster is a terrific cleaner! I use it for just about everything: scouring sinks, cleaning windows, cleaning counters, washing floors, laundry boosting, as a dishwashing machine booster, as a refrigerator cleaner, and removing stuck or burned-on food to pots and pans. It is a natural mineral and is only about $3 a box at my grocery store.

WHITE VINEGAR

White vinegar kills more germs than bleach. It is also great for removing mildew, stains, and grease. White vinegar also whitens laundry. White vinegar can also be inexpensive. I use it (along with borax powder) for so many of my cleaning needs.

HYDROGEN PEROXIDE

There are two hydrogen peroxide products that I know about. One is the type of hydrogen peroxide that you can buy at the pharmacy and the other is food-grade hydrogen peroxide. Food-grade hydrogen peroxide is very strong and needs to be used with caution, and it needs to be stored in the refrigerator after opening. A study was conducted at Virginia Tech on cleaners that kill germs.[153] Hydrogen peroxide in conjunction with vinegar was found to be the most effective, best germ-killing combination. Hydrogen peroxide and vinegar were put in separate spray bottles, and then used separately but together during the same cleaning. One was sprayed (the vinegar or peroxide; it didn't matter which went first), then the other, and then the surface was wiped clean. Hydrogen peroxide is also inexpensive and nontoxic. How can you beat that?!

ALL-PURPOSE WINDOW CLEANER

Combine one-fourth cup white vinegar and one quart of water for a homemade window cleaner. Wear rubber gloves when you are using this, as it can be hard on your skin.

CHAPTER 24

Focus on What You Want to Create

In life, we get what we focus on. If we are always focusing on problems, then we will be getting more problems. So I have found if I always focus on the solution, then I get a much better outcome and life seems easier and more positive.

When you want someone to do something, always focus on what you want to happen, and what you want them to do. They will hear or see what you are saying. If you focus on what you don't want them to do or say "Don't do ___." Then they hear that, but without the *don't*. It is strange how that works, but if you say "Don't run," what they remember is the word "run." Instead, you might say, "Walk, please."

It's not what you *say*; it is what they *hear*. So with children, say what the best outcome can be. "Your homework is always done so quickly and easily, how do you do that?" This puts in the child's mind that this is what they do naturally. They will in turn work that way. When we say things to people, the words carry a lot of energy. Words can be very powerful and can do great good or great harm. Verbal abuse is very painful because it stays with the person in their mind. I think it is the worse form of abuse. It sinks deep into someone's mind and negatively affects them in everything they think about themselves from that time forward. Words can hurt more than physical abuse. When a child is told they are stupid, undeserving, or lazy, they may act accordingly and feel that way for the rest of their lives. What we say to children or other people we love carries great power.

Studying psychosomatic therapy, I have found that this subconscious trauma from verbal abuse can manifest itself in many health-related disorders and illnesses.

When I was raising my children, I always told them they were the smartest, most beautiful, most talented, fabulous children in the world. (In my eyes that was the absolute truth.) Many people told me I shouldn't do that, but I did it anyway. I wanted my children to grow up feeling good about themselves and their abilities. I never wanted them to think they weren't capable of doing anything their hearts desired. They could shoot for the stars. Even if they didn't make the stars, they might make it to the moon of their desires!

I'm glad I told them what I did. Today, my children are happy and successful. I tried my best to give them unconditional love and support every day of their lives. This is the best gift I could give them—it's the best gift we can give anyone we love.

Always focus on what you want to happen and see if things shift to a more positive outcome.

Writing this book has been such a joy for me. I have learned so much over the years and now find so much happiness in being able to share all of this information with you. May you find health and happiness with your children and your family, and have a joyful, healthy lifestyle!

Bless you.

And remember:

The main ingredient is always love!

About the Author

Growing up, Nancy and her three sisters took turns helping their mother— a "scratch" cook—prepare dinner every evening. Their mother would stand at the stairs and call upward in her soprano voice, "Lady in the Kitchen." That's how Nancy learned how to prepare food, plan a meal menu, set a table, and store food properly. Nancy sees her mother still teaching—helping her grandchildren learn these skills.

This certified health counselor and practitioner has claimed her expertise in countless ways. In addition to writing *How to Be a Healthy Vegetarian* and co-authoring *Alive and Cooking: An Easy Guide To Health For You and Your Parents*, Nancy has been:

- certified by Columbia University and the Institute of Integrative Nutrition as a health counselor
- certified by the American Association of Drugless Practitioners as a health practitioner
- certified by Cornell University and the T. Colin Campbell Foundation in plant-based nutrition
- certified for Basic Intensive in Health-Supportive Cooking at the Natural Gourmet Institute for Food and Health in New York City
- certified in psychosomatic therapy with the Australasian Institute of Body-Mind Analysis and Psychosomatic Therapy
- certified raw food chef, instructor, and teacher.

Nancy studied Mediterranean cooking in Syros, Greece, with Australasian College of Health and Sciences. She studied detoxification with Natalia Rose and also studied conscious organic farming and raw food cuisine at the Tree of Life. Nancy is a graduate of Hollins College.

With her all-grade-level teacher's certification for the state of Texas, Nancy taught art, drama, homemaking, and woodshop at a school for children with Learning Differences. In addition, she has taught classes on nutrition and cooking at various places in Texas. She has been affiliated with the United Nations (New York City 2005-2006) and Highland Park Arts Board in Dallas, Texas (1994-2000). Her outreach over the years has been extensive. As associate program director for the non-profit Greater Caribbean Energy and Environment Foundation of Texas, Nancy assists with fundraising and education programs on environmental sustainability of the oceans and ecosystems. She is an award-winning writer, artist, and photographer

This expert counsels clients on nutrition, health, and food preparation one-on-one, in workshops, and at speaking engagements. Nancy is a member of the National Speakers Association. She has been a columnist for the *Park Cities News* and is presently a columnist for *Celebration Magazine* as well as being featured on numerous television and radio programs. Her YouTube channel and website, www.organichealthylifestyle.com, show many of her appearances.

Like her own mother, Nancy taught her children to make meals, plant their organic garden, and volunteer at the Lighthouse for the Blind. (Nancy was Volunteer of the Year and was featured in the United Way Brochure.) She also volunteered at White Bridle Horse Humane Society and was a docent at the Dallas Zoo. She is presently a certified licensed wildlife rehabilitator in the state of Texas and volunteers with the DFW Wildlife Coalition.

Nancy's two children received scholarships at the University of Texas Law School. Today, her son Gibbons (who attended Louisiana State University undergraduate school on an academic scholarship) is a trial lawyer with a Louisiana firm doing environmental and commercial litigation. While finishing her law school degree, her daughter Amanda is working with the Office of the Co-Prosecutors at the United Nations Assistance to the Khmer Trials at the Extraordinary Chambers in the Courts of Cambodia, in Phnom Penh. She is building cases against leaders of the Khmer Rouge for war crimes. Previously, Amanda spent two years with the Peace Corps in Mali, Africa. There, she raised money and helped build an adult literacy center.

Recipes at a Glance

Healthy Drinks

Flavors and Sweeteners for Alternative Milks

Meals for Everyone—Great Baby Foods

Breakfast Foods

Soups

Main Dishes

Side Dishes

Recipes: Vegan, Vegetarian, Raw, Gluten-Free

Teas, Juices, Drinks: Vegan/Vegetarian/Raw/Gluten-free

Non-Dairy Milks: Vegan/Vegetarian/Raw/Gluten-free

Baby Foods: Vegan/Vegetarian/Gluten-free

Desserts: Vegetarian/Gluten-free Recipes

Desserts: Vegetarian/Raw/Gluten-free Recipes

Remedies: Vegan/Vegetarian/Raw/Gluten-free

Remedies: Vegetarian/Raw/Gluten-free

Resources

Following are an array of wonderful resources I use and have found to be extremely helpful. It includes items from grocery stores to brands of gluten-free and whole grain pastas. I hope they will help you, too.

AIR DECONTAMINATION MACHINES

Odorox

www.organichealthylifestyle.com

This machine puts out a high chemical-free HO, over 15 on a PH scale, which is able to clean odors, mold, virus, bacteria, and fungi out of the air as well as on soft and hard surfaces. If anyone in your family has breathing problems, this machine will benefit them. It makes the air more bio-available and safer to breathe. It is great for removing odor (such as toxic remodeling odor or pet odor). It comes in both portable and in duct systems. They are made in Florida. They are built to last 20 years. This air machine is so incredible I became a distributor. Contact me for more information: Nancy@organichealthylifestyle.com.

ALTERNATIVE AND MEDICAL HEALING INSTITUTES

Optimum Health Institute

www.optimumhealth.org/locations/ohi-austin.htm

Found in two locations, California and Texas.

Tree of Life Rejuvenation Center

treeofliferejuvenationcenter.wordpress.com/
tree-of-life-rejuvenation-center/

The Hippocrates Institute

secure.hippocratesinst.org

Gerson Institiute
http://gerson.org/gerpress/clinics/

Tennant Institute for Integrative Medicine
www.tennantinstitute.us
Dr. Tennant works in all kinds of healing modalities, but he is one of the few surgeons to be awarded the Corboy Award for Contributions to Ophthalmology and the Recognition Award from the American Academy of Ophthalmology. He works in many types of healing modalities.

Dr. David Brownstein M.D.
Dr. David Brownstein M.D.is an internationally recognized physician who has a clinic. He is a leading expert in thyroid disorders.
www.dr.brownstein.com

Tenpenny Integrative Medical Center
www.tenpennyimc.com
Dr. *Sherri J. Tenpenny*
Dr. Tenpenny, M.D. is an internationally recognized physician and author, who has a medical center. She is a leading expert on immunizations.
7380 Engle Rd, Middleburg Heights, OH 44130
(440) 239-3438

Dr. Johanna Budwig
www.budwigcenter.com
Dr. Budwig was one of Germany's top biochemists as well one of the best cancer researchers throughout all of Europe.

Dr. Tony Jimenez M.D.
Hope 4 Cancer
Dr. Tony Jimenez M.D. is an internationally recognized physician who has a clinic to diagnose, prevent, and treat cancer patients.
www.hope4cancer.com

Dr. Francisco Contreras, M.D.
Oasis Of Hope
Dr. Francisco Contreras, M.D. is an internationally recognized physician who has a clinic to diagnose, prevent, and treat cancer patients.
www.oasisofhope.com

Stanislaw R. Burzynski, M.D., PhD
www.burzynskiclinic.com
Dr. Burzynski is an internationally recognized physician and bio-chemical researcher who has a clinic to diagnose, prevent, and treat cancer patients.

Dr. Nicholas Gonzalez, M.D.
Dr. Nicholas Gonzalez, M.D.is an internationally recognized physician, scientist and author, who has a clinic to diagnose, prevent, and treat cancer patients.
www.dr-gonzalez.com

Dr. Lawrence B. Palevsky, MD, F.A.A.P.
www.drpalevsky.com or contact info@drpalevsky.com
Dr. Palevsky is a board-certified pediatrician who received his medical degree from the NYU School of Medicine in 1987, completed it at The Mount Sinai Hospital in NYC in 1990, and served as a pediatric fellow in the ambulatory care out-patient department at Bellevue Hospital in NYC. Part of Dr. Palevsky's experience and research concerns: vaccination, immunizations, and their effects on children and the lack of studies that have been done to prove they are necessary and/or safe.

Dr. Palevsky is a Fellow of the American Academy of Pediatrics, co-founder and president of the Holistic Pediatric Association (www.hpakids.org) and past president of the American Holistic Medical Association (www.holisticmedicine.org). He is located in Northport, Long Island and Manhattan, NYC.

Dr. Palevsky offers consultations and educational programs to families and practitioners in preventive and holistic health; vaccination controversies; childhood development; lifestyle changes; nutrition for adults, infants and children; safe, alternative treatments for common and difficult to treat acute and chronic pediatric and adult conditions; mindful parenting; and rethinking the medical paradigm.

Joseph Mercola, MD, interviewed Dr. Palevsky addressing immunizations. See "Expert Pediatrician Exposes Vaccine Myths"
http://articles.mercola.com/sites/articles/archive/2009/11/14/expert-pediatrician-exposes-vaccine-myths.aspx

ALTERNATIVE AND MEDICAL HEALING PRACTITIONERS

Dr. Michael W. Hall, DC, CCST, DABCN, FIACN & Dr. Cara Hall, DC

www.hallchiropracticwellnesscenter.chiromatrixbase.com
972-304–3900
Dr. Michael Hall is a chiropractic neurologist. With his wife, Dr. Cara Hall, DC, who is also a chiropractor trained in clinical neurology and therapeutic massage, they run the Hall Chiropractic and Family Wellness Center in Dallas and in Coppell, Texas.

Nancy Addison CHC, AADP
Nutrition & Health Counseling
Healthful Cooking & Raw Food Chef & Instructor
nancy@organichealthylifestyle.com
www.nancyaddison.com
214-202-9243

Cynthia Champion-Olson ND, CN, CTN
drc4health@msn.com
760-471-2625

Dr. Sandra Bontemps, DC
649 U.S. 1, North Palm Beach, FL 33408
561-845-2300

Dr. Mary Warren
Chiropractor
214-363-3377
www.vitalforcewellness.com

Dr. Elizabeth Naylor
Holistic Health Practitioner
Hair analysis
elizabethnaylor@ebenezerwellness.com

Dr. Alan Chen DC
Acupuncture
He is a fourteenth generation Chinese Medical Doctor.
4100 W 15th St Ste 116
Plano, TX 75093
(972) 599-0852 (Office)

Dr. Bill Osmunson DDS, MPH
Comprehensive Dentist using preventative and the least invasive biological options.
bill@teachingsmiles.comBILLOSMUBeavertobill@teachingsmiles.com

Dr. Daniel Strader DDS
Biological Dentist – non-toxic dentist
8222 Douglas Ave.
Dallas, TX 75225
214-363-7777

BLENDERS AND JUICERS

Breville Juicer
www.compare99.com/p/Breville-Juicers?p2=Juicers&gclid=CL2Zl9yalasCFVsS2godTQF5mw
This juicer is easy to use and pretty easy to clean as well. It is also comparatively low-priced. The Breville Juice Fountain boasts several features that other popular juice extractor brands don't have at good prices.

Vitamix
secure.vitamix.com/?COUPON=06-006525&store=1
I love this product so much, I became an affiliate.

Blendtec
www.blendtec.com
This blender is easy to clean, powerful, and great for liquefying any food.

Lexen Juicers
www.lexenproducts.com

Discount Juicers
www.discountjuicers.com
Discount Juicers has a large selection of juicers for wheatgrass and various other fruits and vegetables, which often need different juicers for juicing. Some are manual and some are electric. The site has some information about the different juicers, and rates them.

BREADS AND PASTA

Food For Life
www.foodforlife.com
This company, makes products are crafted in the likeness of the Holy Scripture verse Ezekiel 4:9 to ensure unrivaled honest nutrition and pure, delicious flavors. Ezekiel 4:9 Breads are delicious.

Alvarado Street Bakery
www.alvaradostreetbakery.com/index.html
This company makes delicious organic whole-grain breads. Outside of California, its breads can be found in the freezer section of the market. Located north of San Francisco in Sonoma County, its products are sold in the United States, Canada, and Japan.

One Degree Organic Foods
www.veganic.com
Organic, sprouted grain Breads with seeds.

Doctor Kracker

www.drkracker.com

This company features organic whole-grain crackers in a variety of flavors.

Mary's Gone Crackers

www.marysgonecrackers.com

These crackers are organic, kosher, non-GMO, whole-grain, vegan, and wheat-free. They contain no hydrogenated oils and are manufactured in a gluten-free, dairy-free, nut-free facility.

Wholly Wholesome

www.whollywholesome.com

This company makes organic whole wheat or spelt pie crust shells.

Wanda's – Nature Farm Foods.

www.heartlandgourmet.net/organicmixes.html

I know them as Wanda's Bread Mixes. Homemade bread is a fabulous way to make your home smell fabulous! Here is my favorite bread company that sells bread mixes. You can use them with a bread machine. If you order a large amount, you can get a price break.

I like to buy the 10-grain bread mix that's organic. It's fabulous!

Rice and Pasta

www.lundberg.com

Lundberg offers organic whole brown rice pasta- vegan- gluten-free. It's easy and delicious. Be careful not to overcook the pasta.

Tinkyana Rice Pasta

www.nextag.com/tinkyada-rice-pasta/compare-html?nxtg=7c750a24051b-CF63729B7EA53C31

This brand is very good for gluten-free pasta. It's made from certified organic whole-grain rice and does not become mushy when cooked, if you don't cook it too long.

Bionaturae
www.bionaturae.com
This is a resource for whole-grain, certified organic pasta.

DeBoles Organic and All-Natural Pastas
www.deboles.com
My daughter and I love the spelt pasta.

Annie's Organic
www.Annies.com
My kids love the shells with real aged cheddar. Though some of their products are made with whole-grain ingredients, others are not. Annie's also makes other products, but read the ingredient label carefully and check for the whole grain and sugar content.

Blue Mountain Organics
www.bluemountainorganics
This company sells raw, sprouted, organic, phytic free flour, seeds, grains, granolas, etc.

BODY CARE PRODUCTS

Young Living Essential Oils
I love these products. I use the thieves mouthwash, toothpaste, hand sanitizer and the thieves cleaning liquids. They are fantastic.
https://www.youngliving.org/nancyaddison

NYR Organics

https://us.nyrorganic.com/shop/NancyAddison/area/shop-online
Certified organic makeup, body care, baby care, and essential oils.
If you have a health business, you can become a distributor. I love this product so much, I became a distributor.

Jusuru

www.jusuru.com

Bio cell liquid is a revolutionary liquid nutraceutical that promotes healthy aging, active joints, and young-looking skin. It even tastes great! It helps with cellular regeneration. It does amazing things for helping rid the body of joint pain, eczema, dry skin, joint mobility and much more. Their pet and equine blend are also phenomenal. This is my fountain of youth secret weapon.

The name Jusuru comes from the Japanese word meaning "to live!" Its ingredients are all natural. I love the way it makes me look and feel! I also use their skin care line.

I take Jusuru liquid bio cell product for my joints and my skin. This product has seven international patents and has had 37 clinical trials. The sports liquid is NSF approved.

I also use the company's skin care products. Together, they have helped my skin become smoother and my joints become more limber and less painful. As a representative (rep #220555), I would love to help you get your wholesale account and show you how to use these products in the most optimum way possible. Email me at Nancy@organichealthylifestyle.com and let me know if you want more information.

BATH PRODUCTS

Iodine-Magnetic Clay Baths

www.magneticclay.com

Nancy's Sea Salts
www.organichealthylifeststyle.com
nancy@organichealthylifestyle.com
Nancy's Sea Salts are bath salts that help the body detox from radiation.

BOOKS BY TITLE

ABC of Asthma, Allergies and Lupus: Eradicate Asthma—Now! by Dr. Fereydoon Batmanghelidj
Alive and Cooking by Maryann De Leo and Nancy Addison
Alkalize or Die by Dr. Theodore A. Baroody
Anatomy of the Spirit by Caroline Myss, PhD
The Anti-Inflammation Zone by Dr. Barry Sears
Blink by Malcolm Gladwell
The Cancer Solution by Robert Willner, MD, PhD
Candida Albicans: Could Yeast Be Your Problem? by Leon Chaitow, ND, DO
The China Study by T. Colin Campbell, PhD
Coconut Cures by Bruce Fife, ND
Complete Candida Yeast Guidebook: Everything You Need to Know About Prevention, Treatment & Diet, Revised 2nd Edition by Jeanne Marie Martin and Zoltan P. Rona, MD
Daylight Robbery: The Importance of Sunlight to Health by Dr. Damien Downing
Diet for a New America by John Robbins
Eat, Drink and Be Healthy by Walter C. Willett, MD
Enzyme Nutrition: The Food Enzyme Concept by Dr. Edward Howell
Enzymes for Health and Longevity by Dr. Edward Howell
Excitotoxins: The Taste That Kills by Dr. Russell L. Blaylock
Fast Food Nation by Eric Schlosser
Food and Healing by Annemarie Colbin
Food for Life by Neal Barnard, MD
The Food Revolution by John Robbins

Foods That Fight Pain by Neal Barnard, MD
Genetic Roulette by Jeffrey Smith
Heal Your Body by Louise L. Hay
Healing with Whole Foods by Paul Pritchard
Health and Nutrition Secrets That Can Save Your Life by Dr. Russell L. Blaylock
The Hippocrates Diet and Health Program by Dr. Ann Wigmore
How to be a Healthy Vegetarian by Nancy Addison
How to Deal With Back Pain and Rheumatoid Joint Pain by Dr. Fereydoon Batmanghelidj
Light, Radiation and You: How to Stay Healthy by John Ott
Listen from the Inside Out: An Everyday Guide to the Secrets of Sound Healing by Sharon Carne
Living on Live Food by Alissa Cohen
The McDougall Program for a Healthy Heart: A Live-Saving Approach to Preventing and Treating Heart Disease by John A. McDougall, MD; recipes by Mary McDougall
The Message from Water by Masaru Emoto
The Natural Hygiene Handbook by the American Natural Hygiene Society
Natural Strategies for the Cancer Patient by Dr. Russell Blaylock
Obesity Cancer & Depression: Their Common Cause & Natural Cure by Dr. Fereydoon Batmanghelidj
Prescription for Nutritional Healing: A Practical A–Z Reference to Drug-Free Remedies Using Vitamins, Minerals, Herbs & Food Supplements, 3rd Edition by Phyllis A. Balch, CNC
Program for Reversing Heart Disease: The Only System Scientifically Proven to Reverse Heart Disease Without Drugs or Surgery by Dr. Dean Ornish
Raw: The Uncook Book by Juliano
The Raw Food Detox Diet by Natalia Rose

Raw Food for Everyone: Essential Techniques and 300 Simple-to-Sophisticated Recipes by Alissa Cohen with Leah J. Dubois

The Secret Life of Water by Masaru Emoto

Saying No To Vaccines: A Resource For All Ages by Dr. Sherri Tenpenny D.O.

Skinny Bitch and Skinny Bastard by Rory Freedman and Kim Barnouin

Staying Healthy with Nutrition: The Complete Guide to Diet and Nutritional Medicine by Elson M. Haas, MD

The Sunfood Diet Success System by David Wolfe

There Is a Cure for Diabetes by Gabriel Cousens, MD

Water: For Health, for Healing, for Life: You're Not Sick, You're Thirsty! by Dr. Fereydoon Batmanghelidj

Water Crystal Healing by Masaru Emoto

Water Cures: Drugs Kill: How Water Cured Incurable Diseases by Dr. Fereydoon Batmanghelidj

You Can Heal Your Life by Louise L. Hay

You'll See it When You Believe It by Dr. Wayne Dyer

Your Body's Many Cries for Water by Dr. Fereydoon Batmanghelid

CLEANSING PRODUCTS

Celebrity Cleanse

I (Nancy) use a cleanse that is non-GMO, organiz, raw, vegan, and has gluten-free versions. It can help people detox safely and efficiently. People can lose from 5 to 20 pounds on the 10-day cleanse. It was developed for celebrities and Olympic athletes who needed to maintian their energy, health, and weaight. It has a money-back guarantee. I use the protein shake and supplements as a regular part of my diet.

Contact me (Nancy) if you are interested in trying this cleanse.
nancy@organichealthylifestyle.com or (214) 202-9243

Detox & Cleanse

www.detox.net.au/articles/detoxification.html

Yerba Prima

www.yerba.com

Dr. John Douillard

http://www.lifespa.com

This doctor is a great source for natural health Ayurveda products and news.

He has special cleanse programs at his clinic/spa and on his website.

EMF (Electro Magnetic Field) PROTECTION-

Suggested reading: Bioinitiative about the problem with electromagnetic fields.

This is a excellent report on the problem with the electromagnetic fields.

http://www.bioinitiative.org/

SENERGY

This company has devices where you can measure you EMF in your environment. They also have devices that can help lessen the EMF in your environment.

http://www.senergy.us/

LESS EMF

http://www.lessemf.com/computer.html

Defend Pad

www.defenderpad.com

CELL PHONE PROTECTION

I highly recommend using a case for your cell phone that cuts down on the radiation.

I use this one. I also use protection for my laptop and my home.

Silver Shield Cell Phone Case
https://silvershield.com/

ENZYMES AND VITAMINS
Buy vitamins made with whole, organic food.
The body reads whole food much better than it reads isolated chemicals.

Dr. Mercola Digestive Enzymes
products.mercola.com/digestive-enzymes
Dr. Mercola has many other healthful products on his website and a great newsletter.

Innate GTF Chromium
www.7lights.net
A whole food natural chromium vitamin supplement.
Chromium helps carry the glucose from the blood into the muscles.

Manna Bears
www.mannatech.com
Chewy gummy bear type of supplement for children

Floradil Multivitamins
These are made of whole food ingredients, which the body "reads" this better than isolated chemicals combinations.

Panacea Multivitamin
www.panacea4u.com
A mineral and superfood supplement

Garden of Life
www.gardenoflife.com
A variety of whole-food-based and organic products;
They have a phytase digestive enzyme.
I love this product so much, I became a distributor.

New Chapter Organics
www.newchapter.com
A variety of whole-food-based and organic products

Ancient Minerals
www.magneticclay.com
Ultra-pure magnesium oil

Organic Sulfur Crystals Supplement
www.7lights.net

HEALTHFUL COOKING SCHOOLS

The Natural Gourmet Institute
naturalgourmetinstitute.com/
48 W. 21st St., 2nd Floor
New York, NY 10010
(212) 645–5170

The Natural Gourmet Institute offers a variety of classes on health, supportive culinary arts, and theory year-round to the public. It also has a wonderful chef-training program.

Natural Epicurean Academy of Culinary Arts
www.naturalepicurean.com
1700 S Lamar Blvd

Austin, TX 78704
(512) 476-2276
The Natural Epicurean offers a comprehensive professional chef training program that focuses on the theory and practice. I've taught nutrition classes there.

HOME DELIVERY OF ORGANIC FOODS

Look for local co-ops in your area, a great resource for local, fresh, organic food.

Greenling

www.greenling.com
Greenling delivers foods to your home in certain areas. It is terrific.

KITCHEN SUPPLIES

Williams-Sonoma

www.williams-sonoma.com/
This store has a good selection of high-quality kitchen tools and equipment.

Sur la Table

www.surlatable.com
This store offers a good selection of high-quality kitchen tools and equipment.

Real Goods

www.realgoods.com/product/09-9115.do
It provides recycled and PBA-free containers, also plastic bowls.

MAIL-ORDER FOODS

Natalia Rose/Detox the World

www.detoxtheworld.com/

Located in New York City, Natalia sells food for delivery just about anywhere. She has resources for juicing, detoxing, colonics, etc. as well as great books and recipes. Her site is an awesome resource.

Veggie Brothers

www.veggiebrothers.com 1-877-834-2655

For vegetarian cooking, this is an online vegan/vegetarian store that has the freshest natural and organic ingredients available. None of their ingredients has been genetically modified.

- 100% organic
- 100% wheat and gluten-free
- Single portions are 10.5 oz.
- Sides are 3.5-5 oz.
- Soups are 9 oz.
- There are 2-4 servings with each appetizer.

Raw Guru

www.rawguru.com/store/raw-food/nama-shoyu-raw-organic-

This site lets you order raw food online.

Local Harvest

www.localharvest.org

Organic Authority

www.organicauthority.com

This website can help you locate locally grown organic foods.

MAIL-ORDER FOODS ALSO IN HEALTH FOOD/GROCERY STORES

Organic Healthy Lifestyle / Nancy Addison

www.nancyaddison.com

http://www.organichealthylifestyle.com

In the store on this website (my own website), I sell products that have improved my health. There, you can purchase unrefined sea salt products, mouthwash, vitamins, organic body lotions, essential oils, my books, cooking DVDs, audio recordings of my lectures or cooking lessons, Blue Mountain Organic products, Garden of Life Products, organic body care and make up, and more. Nancy@organichealthylifestyle.com

Blue Mountain Organics

http://bluemountainorganics.com

This company sells raw, sprouted phytic acid, grains, flours, baking products.

Go Raw

www.goraw.com

This company has sprouted, organic, sunflower, pumpkin, flax and watermelon seeds and seed bars, sprouted granolas and sprouted grain cookies.

Nuts Online

www.nutsonline.com

This company has raw, organic nuts and seeds.

Eden Foods

www.edenfoods.com/store

This is an organic company owned by the family that started it. The products are made with integrity, and I love their taste and flavor.

18 Rabbits

www.18rabbits.com

This company has high integrity and quality products that are low in added sugar.

They make wonderful granola, food bars, etc. I love them.

Navitas Naturals

www.navitasnaturals.com

This company makes all kinds of wonderful superfood products—superfood supplements, smoothie blends, snacks, and dehydrated coconut water.

Pacific Foods

www.pacificfoods.com

This company sells soups that are low in sugar—a good option for anyone with diabetes—although some flavors are high in sugar. Be sure to read ingredient lists. I like the almond milk (unsweetened vanilla).

Fig Food Company

figfood.com

This company has a variety of products including Tuscan white bean soup, which only has 1 gram of sugar. It provides BPA-free packaging.

Amy's

www.amys.com

Amy's offers a variety of frozen meals and foods. Amy's cheese pizza is delicious. I served it when my children had slumber parties and times when I needed fast, easy, and healthy food for more "mainstream" people. Amy's also has burgers and other meat alternatives. Although this brand is not totally organic and uses soy, it's good to have if you're craving transition food from being a carnivore. I take the Texas Burger when I go to a cookout.

Seeds of Change

www.seedsofchange.com

This company makes wonderful, high quality, organic food products.

Tru Roots

www.truroots.com

This company has a variety of products including sprouted whole grains in bulk.

Shiloh Farms

www.shilohfarms.com

Shiloh Farms is a good brand for bulk organic whole grains.

Bob's Red Mill

www.bobsredmill.com

Bob's Red Mill is carried at most healthy grocery stores along with a variety of healthy grains and flours.

Arrowhead Mills

www.arrowheadmills.com

This company has a variety of products including organic oat bran.

Food for Life

www.foodforlife.com

Its almond Ezekiel 4.9 Sprouted Whole Grain Cereal is one of my favorites along with a delicious variety of breads.

Tapioca

www.edwardandsons.com

This company offers tapioca, certified organic and granulated by Let's Do Organic.

Product of France

Sun Warrior

www.sunwarrior.com/products/sunwarrior-ormusgreens

Sun Warrior makes power-packed, raw, and organic green concentrated food powder as well as protein powders.

Sensational Sea Salt Seasoning

www.organichealthylifestyle.com

Nancy@organichealthylifestyle.com

Sensational Sea Salt Seasoning was created by Nancy Addison (me!). This proprietary seasoning blend of mineral and nutrient dense, whole, raw, organic food is made of the finest sea salts, sea kelps, and omega 3, and vitamin E-rich seeds to boost the absorption of iodine, the main nutrient that supports the thyroid gland. Use in place of normal salt. Yes, this is my sea salt seasoning, and it's delicious!

Sensational Sea Salt: Unrefined Sea Salt

www.organichealthylifestyle.com

I also have a plain, nutrient-dense unrefined, fine-grained sea salt that's naturally high in iron, iodine, potassium, magnesium as well as other minerals. Check out Sensational Sea Salts, Bolivian Rose Salt, Sexy Sea Salt (bath salts that help the body detox from radiation) at Nancy@organichealthylifestyle.com

Organic Ville Foods

organicvillefoods.com/products/condiments/stone-ground-organic-mustard

This is a good source for organic stone-ground mustard.

Hain Safflower Mayonnaise

www.hainpurefoods.com/index.php

SweetLeaf
www.sweetleaf.com
1203 W. San Pedro St.
Gilbert, AZ 85233 (800) 899–9908
Makers of SweetLeaf Sweetener®, a source for stevia (sugar alternative).

Now
www.nowfoods.com
This company provides a brand of xylitol.

Gold Mine Natural Food Co.
www.goldminenaturalfood.com
Nama Shoyu raw, organic soy sauce is raw, organic, non-genetically modified, and aged four years.

Braggs Soy Sauce
www.bragg.com
Braggs makes wonderful organic soy sauce and apple cider vinegar as well as other products.

Teeccino Caffé, Inc.
teeccino.com/category/11/Herbal-Coffees.html
P.O. Box 40829
Santa Barbara, CA 93140 (800) 498–3434
(805) 966–0999 (outside the U.S. and Canada)
This coffee provides coffee alternatives.

Garden of Life: Vitamins, Protein Powders, Green Food Powders
www.organichealthylifestyle.com or www.gardenoflife.com
Garden of Life has vitamins, snack bars, green foods, meal substitutes, and protein powders that are raw, certified organic, gluten-free, and vegan.

Pomona's Universal Pectin

www.pomonapectin.com

This is what I use to make Jell-O-type foods. Recipes can be found on the box.

Purity Farms

www.purityfarms.com

Organic ghee

Living Harvest

www.livingharvest.com (888) 690–3958

Hemp oil

Essential Living Foods

www.essentiallivingfoods.com

Cacao powder

Ultimate Superfoods

www.ultimatesuperfoods.com

Water Purifiers

http://www.lifeionizer.com/nourishingwater/nourishingwater

This is a great place to purchase all types of water purifiers, alkalizers, and shower heads.

Food-Grade Hydrogen Peroxide

www.narualzing.com

This Natural Zing hydrogen peroxide cleans fruits and vegetables. I use this brand a lot. (Keep it safely out of reach of children.)

ORGANIZATIONS AND PROGRAMS

Institute of Integrative Nutrition

http://www.integrativenutrition.com/
iinbook?erefer=0015000000IyQPEAA3

This school teaches holistic nutrition that helps integrate mainstream medical philosophy with holistic healing. Download two chapters of this book.

Physicians Committee for Responsible Medicine

www.pcrm.org
5100 Wisconsin Ave. NW, Suite 404
Washington, DC 20016 (202) 686–2210

I joined this committee before I was a vegetarian and found it to be an amazing source of information on promoting preventative medicine, higher standards of ethics, and effective research. It offers vegetarian starter kits. Dr. Neal Barnard is a part of this organization.

Bee Action

Saving the bees
www.beeaction.org

Food and Water

www.foodandwater.org
389 Rt. 215
Walden, VT 05873 (800) EAT–SAFE

This group provides information on food and water, leading campaigns against toxic and unsafe food and water practices, and helping protect our water.

Food Animal Concerns Trust (FACT)
www.foodanimalconcerns.org
P.O. Box 14599 Chicago, IL 60614 (773) 525–4952
FACT promotes more humane, safe, and sustainable methods of raising livestock and poultry, and runs food safety and on-farm programs.

The Cornucopia Institute
www.cornucopia.org
This Institute seeks economic justice for the family-scale farming community. Through research, advocacy, and economic development, its goal is to empower farmers, partnered with consumers, in support of ecologically produced local, organic, and authentic food.

MOVIES

Roadmap to Healthy Foods in School available from Natural Press 1-877-629-8398.
(This is the story of the Appleton School System that turned itself around using healthier foods in their schools.)

Doctored – a documentary by Working Pictures, a Jeff Hays Film

Forks Over Knives – a documentary by Virgil Films www.forksoverknives.com

Healing Cancer From The Inside Out – a documentary by Mike Anderson

Water, the Great Mystery – a documentary about water

THRIVE is a documentary by Foster and Kimberly Gamble. You can watch it on: www.youtube.com/watch?v=lEV5AFFcZ-s

The Truth About Cancer – a documentary (11 part series) by Ty Bolinger

Origins by Dr. Pedram , a wonderful movie about healing, toxins, our origins, etc.

PROBIOTIC FOODS

Inner-Eco
www.inner-eco.com
A coconut, power-packed probiotic kefir.

High Country
www.highcountrykombucha.com

Happy Herbalist
www.happyherbalist.com/kombucha.htm
Kombucha-making kits

Garden of Life
www.gardenoflife.com
Raw, organic, whole food based products.
Provides a variety of supplements as well as food.

Sunrider
This company has wonderful stevia that is unrefined, detoxification teas, and more.
Contact me at Nancy@organichealthylifestyle.com or Sharyn Wynters at DrWynters@aol.com for more information on these products.

Rice Cooker
www.lotusfoods.com/index.php/products/rice-cookers/

Lotus Foods Rice Cooker and Vegetable Steamer has an inner cooking pot and steaming tray constructed completely of mirror-finish stainless steel.

SEA SALT

Bolivian Rose Sea Salt

www.organichealthylifestyle.com

This unrefined, mineral rich, fine-grained sea salt is naturally high in iron, iodine, potassium, magnesium as well as other minerals; it's mined from Bolivia.

Sensational Sea Salt Seasoning

www.sensationalseasalt.com

www.organichealthylifestyle.com

Sensational Sea Salt Seasoning was created by Nancy Addison (me!). This proprietary seasoning blend of mineral and nutrient dense, whole, raw, organic food made up of the finest sea salts, sea kelps, omega 3 and vitamin E-rich seeds to boost the absorption of the iodine, the main nutrient that supports the thyroid gland. Use in place of your normal salt. Yes, this is my sea salt seasoning, and it's delicious!

SEEDS AND SPROUTING SUPPLIES

For a website with a list of organic, sprouted grain and bean growers and resources, go to http://www.greenpeople.org/WholeGrains.htm

Got Sprouts

www.gotsprouts.com

The Hippocrates Health Institute

www.hippocrateshealthinstitute.com

1443 Palmdale Court

West Palm Beach, FL 33411

This is a great resource for seeds, equipment, raw food, vegan food, and a great place to go for healthy rejuvenation of the body.

Probiotics for the Garden, People, and Pets
I use this for cleaning my seeds, feeding my garden, composting, and flea prevention for my pets. It is used by the SPCA for flea prevention in a natural way.

Seeds of Change
www.seedsofchange.com
This is my favorite place to purchase seeds. The company has organic gardening seeds and makes wonderful, high-quality organic food products.

Sprouting Seeds
http://organicsproutingseeds.com
TeraGanix, Inc. (formerly EM America)
www.teraganix.com
These are probiotics for the earth—the exclusive distributor of Dr. Higa's Effective Microorganisms.

SNACK BARS

Raw Crunch Bars
rawcrunchbar.myshopify.com
These are great for food on the go and come in cranberry, chocolate, goji berry, and blueberry.

Wild Bar
www.wildbar.info
Gluten-free, vegan, kosher

SOAPS AND CLEANING PRODUCTS

Dr. Bronner's Magic Soap

www.drbronner.com (760) 743–2211

This is a blend of pure castille soap. Some contain essential oils. I buy them in large bottles and use them to refill my hand soap containers.

Oxo Brite

www.ecos.com

This non-toxic stain remover is used on almost all of my stains. I put a scoop or two in a bowl of water and soak my stained clothing overnight. It really brightens white, too.

Twenty Mule Team Borax

www.20muleteamlaundry.com

One of the best all-purpose cleaners, it's a natural mineral and inexpensive. You won't believe how great this is!

Young Living Oils

I love these products. I have used them for over 20 years.

I use their Thieves mouthwash, cleaning liquids, non-toxic hand sanitizer and wipes, etc.

www.youngliving.org/nancyaddison

SPICES

Frontier Natural Products

www.frontiercoop.com

Mountain Rose Company
www.mountainroseherbs.com

STORES

Whole Foods Market
www.wholefoodsmarket.com

This is my favorite store for grocery shopping. They were the first nationally certified organic grocer in the United States. I understand it tries hard to keep quality at the most optimum level, and that it stands by its products with a wonderful return policy.

Whole Foods Market also has its 365 brand products, which are usually less expensive than other products. I asked an employee about the 365 products that are not labeled organic. She researched it and told me that Whole Foods Market makes every attempt to use only non–genetically modified foods in all of their products, if at all possible. Whole Foods has locations in the United States, Canada, and United Kingdom.

Central Market
www.CentralMarket.com/Home.aspx
This is a Texas store that's expanding. It offers mail order, cooking classes, and a variety of other services.

Sprouts
www.sprouts.com
This store sells organic produce and products. Based in Arizona, it has stores in California, Texas, Colorado, and Arizona.

Natural Grocers
www.naturalgrocers.com
This store sells organic produce and products, often at great prices. This store sells refrigerated raw nuts. Nuts turn rancid quickly, so they must be refrigerated. I buy my nuts at this store. It has locations in Idaho, Kansas,

Missouri, Nebraska, New Mexico, Oklahoma, Texas, Utah, and Wyoming.

New Frontiers
newfrontiersmarket.com
This store is a supporter of non-genetically modified foods. I have found nice organic produce and products at this market. It has locations in Arizona and California.

Green Grocer
www.greengrocerdallas.com/
This healthy grocery store is in Dallas and Chicago. It doesn't carry GMO (genetically engineered) foods. I love that!

Trader Joes
www.traderjoes.com
Trader Joes carries some organic produce and products. Its private label food is from non-genetically modified sources.

TEAS

Organic India
www.organicindia.com
For a brand of tulsi tea.

Yogi Tea
www.yogiproducts.com
Good selection of organic teas.

Mountain Rose Herbs
www.mountainroseherbs.com
An amazing selection of rare teas, herbs, oils, information, etc.

Celestial Seasonings Tea
www.celestialseasonings.com

GT's Kombucha Tea
www.GTSkombucha.com (877) RE-Juice
Organic, raw kombucha (lightly effervescent fermented drink of sweetened black tea)

References

Adams, Mike. "CDC Adjusts Fluoride Poisoning of America's Water Supply to a Lower Level." Natural News website. www.naturalnews.com/030952_CDC_fluoride.html.

"Cities Fluoridating Drinking Water with Toxic Chemicals." NewsTarget.com website. March 31, 2005. www.newstarget.com/005900.htm.

"Agriculture Fact Book 98." US Department of Agriculture website. www.usda.gov/news/pubs/fbook98/ch1a.htm.

"Alert: Protein Drinks: You Don't Need the Extra Protein or the Heavy Metals Our Tests Found." *Consumer Reports* website. www.consumerreports.org/cro/magazine-archive/2010/july/food/protein-drinks/overview/index.htm.

American Society for Microbiology.

Anderson, ND, NMD, Dr. Richard. *Cleanse and Purify Thyself Volume 1, Revised Edition* (Avery Trade, 1991).

Cleanse and Purify Thyself Volume 2, Revised Edition. Avery Trade, 1998.

Antoniou, Michael, Paul Brack, Andrés Carrasco, John Fagan, and Mohamed Habib. "GM Soy. Sustainable? Responsible?" GMWatch website. www.gmwatch.org/files/GMsoy_Sust_Respons_SUMMARY_ENG_v6.pdf.

"The Arbor, Alcohol and Drug and Rehab." Detox.net website. www.detox.net.au/articles/detoxification.html.

"Average Mineral Content in Selected Vegetables, 1914–1997." Nutrition Security Institute website. www.nutritionsecurity.org/PDF/Mineral%20Content%20in%20Vegetables.pdf.

Azulay, Sol. International Specialty Supply website. www.sproutnet.com/sprouts_in_the_press.htm.

"There's More to Sprouts than Just a Little Crunch in Your Salad." Interview with *San Diego Earth Times*. November 1997.

Barclay, Eliza. "What's Best for Kids: Bottled Water or Fountains?" National Geographic News, March 3, 2010.

Barnard, MD, Neal. *Food for Life*. Three Rivers Press, 1994.

Barron, Jon. "Myth or Fact: Is Canola Oil Healthy?" Baseline of Health Foundation website. October 9, 2006. www.jonbarron.org/heart-health/bl061009/is-canola-oil-healthy.

Bassler, Dr. Anthony. "A Common Mistake that Prevents Most People from Losing Weight...and How to Avoid It! Why This Simple 'First Step' Should Be Part of Any Weight Management, Anti-Aging and Health Improvement Program." Vegetarian Times, January 2004.

Batmanghelidj, Dr. Fereydoon. *ABC of Asthma, Allergies and Lupus, First Edition*. Global Health Solutions, Inc., 2000.

-*Water: For Health, for Healing, for Life: You're Not Sick, You're Thirsty!* Hachette Digital, Inc., 2003.

-*Your Body's Many Cries for Water, Third Edition.* Global Health Solutions, Inc., 2008.

Bellatti, Andy. "You Ask, I Answer: Soy Protein Isolate." Medpedia website. www.medpedia.com/news_analysis/98-Small-Bites/entries/71677-You-Ask-I-Answer-Soy-Protein-Isolate.

Blaylock, R.L. *Excitotoxins: The Taste that Kills*. Health Press, 1994.

Bolen, Jim. "Histamine/Anti-histamine and the Dangers of Taking Anti-histamine." Water Cure website. www.watercure2.org/histamines.htm.

"Bottled Water: Pure Drink or Pure Hype?" Natural Resources Defense Council website. www.nrdc.org/water/drinking/bw/bwinx.asp.

"A Brief History of Protein, Passion, Social Bigotry, Rats and Enlightenment." *The McDougall Newsletter, Volume 2, Number 12*, December 2003. www.nealhendrickson.com/mcdougall/031200puprotein.htm.

Brock, Dr. Rovenia. Interview with Bob Green on foods that help relieve stress. Oprah Radio. January 1, 2008.

Brownstein, David, M.D. Iodine, *Why You Need It; Why You Can't Live Without It.* 4th edition. Medical Alternatives Press. 2009.

Burry, John N. "More on Preventing Skin Cancer: Author's Reply." *British Medical Journal*, November 23, 2003. www.bmj.com/content/327/7425/1228.1.full.

Campbell, T. Colin, PhD. "Principles of Nutritional Health. Plant-Based Nutrition." eCornell University and T. Colin Campbell Foundation. 2010.

Campbell, T. Colin, PhD. The China Study: *The Most Comprehensive Study of Nutrition Ever Conducted And the Startling Implications for Diet, Weight Loss, and Long-term Health.* BenBella Books. 2006.

Chaitow, Leon. "Candida Albicans: Could Yeast Be Your Problem?" Harvard Gazette website. www.news.harvard.edu/gazette/1997/10.30/GeneticSecretso.html.

"Chemicals in the Environment: Chlorine (CAS NO. 7782-50-5)." Prepared by the Office of Pollution Prevention and Toxics. US Environmental Protection Agency. August 1994.

Cheung, FRCP, Dr. Anthony. "Enzymes." Enerex website. www.enerex.ca/en/articles/digestive-enzymes.

"The 'Chlorinated' Water Issue and the Water Ionization Alternative Using Copper or Silver Nanocrystal Ionization." Biophysica, Inc. website. www.biophysica.com/chlorine.html.

Ciarallo, L., D. Brousseau, and S. Reinert. "Higher-Dose Intravenous Magnesium Therapy for Children with Moderate to Severe Acute Asthma." *Archives of Pediatric & Adolescent Medicine,* October 2000, 154(10): 979–983. National Center for Biotechnology Information website. www.ncbi.nlm.nih.gov/corehtml/pmc/pmcgifs/pmc3_ logo_v5.gif.

Coates, Dr. Wayne. "Chia History." Dr. Wayne Coates's website. www.azchia.com/chia_history.htm.

"Code of Federal Regulations, Title 21, Volume 2." Revised as of April 1, 2009. US Government Printing Office. GPO Access CITE: 21CFR101.22. Pages 72–76.

Cohen, Bryan. "Natural Cures for Enlarged Thyroid." eHow website. www.ehow.com/way_5317305_natural-cures-enlarged-thyroid.html#ixzz1SYtyAarn.

Connett, PhD, Paul. "50 Reasons to Oppose Fluoridation." Canton, N.Y.: St. Lawrence University. Food Consumer website. www.foodconsumer.org/newsite/Non-food/Environment/50_reasons_to_oppose_fluoridation_0109111037.html.

"Consumer Group Calls for Ban on 'Flour Improver': Potassium Bromate Termed a Cancer Threat." Center for Science in the Public Interest website. www.cspinet.org/new/bromate.html.

Cousens, MD, Gabriel. *There Is a Cure for Diabetes*. North Atlantic Books, 2008.

Cromie, William. "Genetic Secrets of Killer Fungus Found." Harvard Gazette website, October 30, 1997. news.harvard.edu/gazette/1997/10.30/ GeneticSecretso.html.

D'Adamo, Dr. Peter J., with Catherine Whitney. "Blood Type O, Food, Beverage and Supplement List." *Eat Right 4 Your Type*. Berkley Books, 1999.

Damato, PhD, Gregory. "GM-Soy: Destroy the Earth and Humans for Profit." Natural News website. May 27, 2009. www.naturalnews.com/026334_soy_Roundup_GMO.html#ixzz1RzIZAWwh.

David, Dr. Donald. "Study suggests nutrient decline in garden crops over past 50 years." Dec. 1, 2004. University of Texas: http://www.utexas.edu/news/2004/12/01/nr_chemistry/ For more information contact Lee Clippard, College of Natural Sciences, 512-232-0675.

Dexter, Beatrice. "Honey and Cinnamon: Mother Nature's Powerful Healing Combination." *Weekly World News*, January 17, 1995. weeklyworldnews.com/archive/.

Diamond, Harvey, and Marilyn Diamond. *Fit for Life II*. The Media Business Publishing, 1985.

"Dietary Supplement Fact Sheet: Calcium." US Office of Diet Supplements, National Institutes of Health website. ods.od.nih.gov/factsheets/Calcium-QuickFacts/.

"Dietary Supplement Fact Sheet: Iron." US Office of Dietary Supplements, National Institutes of Health website. ods.od.nih.gov/factsheets/ iron/.

"Doing it on Your Own: Eating Vegetarian." McGill University website. June 30, 2010. www.mcgill.ca/fitatmcgill/nutrition/doingit/veg/.

Douillard, DC, Dr. John. "Sun Exposure: Don't Be Fooled By Your Sunscreen." Dr. John Douillard's Lifespa.com website. http://lifespa.com/dont-be-fooled-by-your-sunscreen/

- "Vitamin D Has Astonishing Health Benefits." Dr. John Douillard's Lifespa.com website. http://www.lifespa.com/vitamin-d-has-astonishing-health-benefits.

- "Amazing Benefits of Sleeping on Your Left Side." http://lifespa.com/amazing-benefits-of-sleeping-on-your-left-side.

Downing, MB, BS, Dr. Damien. Daylight Robbery: *The Importance of Sunlight to Health*. Arrow Books, 1998.

Dyer, MS, RD, Diana. "What's in Kale? USDA Nutrient Content Data." 365 Days of Kale weblog. February 22, 2009. www.365daysofkale.com/2009/02/whats-in-kale-usda-nutrient-content.html.

Edwards, Michael. "Healthy Sugar Alternatives: Understanding Both Healthy & Not So Healthy Sugars with Their Glycemic Index." Organic Lifestyle magazine, June 12, 2009.

"Effects of microwave radiation on anti-infective factors in human milk." Quan R1, Yang C, Rubinstein S, Lewiston NJ, Sunshine P, Stevenson DK, Kerner JA Jr. *Pediatrics*. 1992. Apr;89(4 Pt 1):667-9.

"Eighty Year Decline in Mineral Content of Medium Apple." Nutrition Security Institute website. www.nutritionsecurity.org/PDF/Mineral%20Content%20of%20One%20Apple.pdf.

El, Dr. Akilah M. "The Health Benefits of Bentonite Clay." Dr. Akilah's website: The Natural Health and Holistic World According to Dr. Akilah El. docakilah.wordpress.com/2011/06/09/the-health- benefits-of-bentonite-clay/.

Emoto, Masuro. *The Hidden Messages in Water*. Atria Books, 2005.

Erasmus, Udo. *Fats That Heal Fats That Kill.* Alive Books, 1993.

Esselstyn, Dr. Caldwell B. Jr. *Prevent and Reverse Heart Disease*. Avery. 2007.

Fallon, Sally, and Mary G. Enig. "Newest Research on Why You Should Avoid Soy." *Nexus magazine, Volume 7, Number 3*, April–May 2000. www.eregimens.com/therapies/Diet/Soy/NewestResearchon-whyYouShouldAvoidSoy.htm.

Fife, ND, Bruce. *Coconut Cures*. Piccadilly Books, Ltd., 1952.

"FoodfromtheRainforests."RainforestActionNetworkwebsite.ran.org/fileadmin/materials/education/factsheets/RAN_RainforestFood.pdf.

Francione, Gary, and Robert Garner. *The Animal Rights Debate: Abolition or Regulation*. Columbia University Press, 2010.

Freedman, Rory, and Kim Barnouin. Skinny Bitch (Running Press, 2005). "From the History of Medicine in the USSR." w3.gorge.net/chriss/kombucha.htm.

Gare, Fran. *The Sweet Miracle of Xylitol*. Basic Health Publications, Inc., 2003.

Garland, Cedric F. "Sun Avoidance Will Increase Incidence of Cancers Overall." *British Medical Journal* website. www.bmj.com/content/327/7425/1228.2.full.

Gittleman, PhD, CNS, Ann Louise. *Get the Sugar Out*. Three Rivers Press, 1996.

Gordon, Dennis. "Vegetable Proteins Can Stand Alone." *Journal of the American Dietetic Association, Volume 96, Issue 3*, March 1996.

Goulart, Frances Sheridan. "Are You Sugar Smart? Linked to Heart Attacks, Kidney Disease, Diabetes and Other Diseases, Sugar Is to the '90s What Cholesterol Was to the '80s—Includes 9 ways to Cope with Sugar Cravings." *American Fitness*, March–April 1991.

Groves, Barry. "Full-Spectrum Sunlight and Cancer: UV Benefits Leukemia and Other Cancers." Second Opinions website. www.second-opinions.co.uk/full_spectrum_sunlight.html.

Guy, RA. "The Diets of Nursing Mothers and Young Children in Peiping." *Chinese Medical Journal*, 1936; 50:434—442.

Haas, Dr. Elson M., with Dr. Buck Levin. *Staying Healthy with Nutrition*. Celestial Arts, 2006.

Hallberg, Leif, Lena Rossander, and Ann-Britt Skanberg. "Phytates and the Inhibitory Effect of Bran on Iron Absorption in Man." *American Journal of Clinical Nutrition, Volume 45*, 1987: 988–996.

Hattersley, Joseph G. "Poisoning by Chlorinated Water." Dr. Joseph Mercola's website. May 1999. articles.mercola.com/sites/articles/archive/2001/01/07/chlorinated-water2.aspx.

"'Healing Clays' Hold Promise in Fight Against MRSA Superbug Infections and Disease." Arizona State University—Biodesign Institute website. April 7, 2008. www.biodesign.asu.edu.

"High-Fructose Corn Syrup: Everything You Wanted to Know, but Were Afraid to Ask." *American Journal of Clinical Nutrition*, December 2008, 88(6):1715S.

Hooper, Rowan. "Top 11 Compounds in US Drinking Water." *New Scientist*, January 12, 2009. www.newscientist.com/article/dn16397-top-11-compounds-in-us-drinking-water.html.

Howell, Dr. Edward. *Enzyme Nutrition*. Avery Publishing Group Inc., 1985.

-*Food Enzymes for Health and Longevity.* Omangod Press, 1980, p. xiii.

-*Intestinal Absorption and Secretion*. E. Skadhange, editor. MTP Press Limited, 1984.

-*Food Enzymes for Health and Longevity, 2nd Edition*. Lotus Press, 1994. Originally published in 1946 as *The Status of Food Enzymes in Digestive and Metabolism*.

"Hunger." FAO news release. September 14, 2010. World Food Programme website. www.wfp.org/hunger/stats,%20FAO%20news%20 release,%2014%20September%202010%20%20source.

Hurrell, Richard, Marcel-A Juillerat, Manju Reddy, Sean Lynch, Sandra Dassenko, and James Cook. "Soy Protein, Phytate, and Iron Absorption in Humans." *American Journal of Clinical Nutrition, Volume 56*, 1992: 573–578.

Hurrell, Richard, Manju Reddy, and James Cook. "Inhibition of Non- Haem Iron Absorption in Man by Polyphenolic-Containing Beverages." *British Journal of Nutrition, Volume 81*, 1999: 289–295.

Hyman, Dr. Mark. "Is Hidden *Fungus* Making You Ill?" Dr. Mark Hyman's website. drhyman.com/is-hidden-fungus-making-you-ill-1737/.

Ilardi, PhD, Stephen. "Dietary Sugar and Mental Illness: A Surprising Link" in *The Depression Cure*. Psychology Today website. www. psychologytoday.com/blog/the-depression-cure/200907/ dietary-sugar-and-mental-illness-surprising-link.

"Inside Information on Important Innovations in Bio-Science and Technology: Liquid 'Stabilized Oxygen'." Bio/Tech News, 2000. www. biotechnews.com/docs/vit-o_prn.html.

Ismail, Baraem, Bradley L. Reuhs, and S. Suzanne Nielsen. "Analysis of Food Contaminants, Residues, and Chemical Constituents of Concern." Seventeenth Report of the Joint FAO/WHO Expert Committee on Food Additives, World Health Organization techn. Rep. Ser. 1974, No. 539; FAO Nutrition Meetings Report Series, 1974, No. 53. World Health Organization, Geneva, 1974. The evaluations contained in this publication were prepared by the Joint FAO/WHO Expert Committee on Food Additives, which met in Geneva, June 25–July 4, 1973.

Jensen, DC, ND, PhD, Dr. Bernard. *Dr. Jensen's Guide to Better Bowel Care: A Complete Program for Tissue Cleansing through Bowel Management*. Avery, 1998.

- *Health Magic Through Chlorophyll from Living Plant Life*. Bi World Industries, Inc.

- *Tissue Cleansing Through Bowel Management*. Self-published, 1980.

Kamen, Betty, PhD, and Michael Rosenbaum, MD. "Microwaved Veggies: Bad News." *Journal of the Science of Food and Agriculture* 2003; 93(14), October 2003.

Katch, Frank I. *History Makers*. www.sportsci.org/news/history/chittenden/chittenden.html.

"Kombucha Health Benefits." Written by "Kristen M." Food Renegade website. www.foodrenegade.com/kombucha-health-benefits/.

"Kombucha Tea." Mayo Clinic website. www.mayoclinic.com/health/kombucha-ea/AN01658.

Kujovich, Jody. "Which Foods Keep the Body From Absorbing Iron from Pills?" Livestrong website. www.livestrong.com/article/280321-which-foods-keep-the-body-from-absorbing-iron-from-iron-pills/.

Leson, Gero, and Petra Pless. *Hemp Foods and Oils for Health.* Hemptech, 1991.

Mangels, PhD, RD, Reed. "Protein in the Vegan Diet." Vegetarian Resource Group website. VRG.org.

Manning, Richard. "The Oil We Eat: Following the Food Chain Back to Iraq." *Harper's*, February 2004.

Martin, Jeanne Marie, and Zoltan P. Rona, MD. *Complete Candida Yeast Guidebook, Everything You Need to Know About Prevention, Treatment & Diet, Revised Edition*. Prima Health, 2000.

Mayo Clinic website. www.mayoclinic.com.

McDougall, MD, John. "Nutrition in the Medical Clinic Part III" lecture. "Plant-Based Nutrition." eCornell University.

McMahon, James P. "Which Bottled Water Is the Best?" Sweetwater LLC website. www.cleanairpurewater.com/best_bottled_water.html.

Mercola, Dr. Joseph. "Everything You HAVE TO KNOW about Dangerous Genetically Modified Foods." Dr. Joseph Mercola's website. October 17, 2009. articles.mercola.com/sites/articles/archive/2009/10/17/ everything-you-have-to-know-about-dangerous-genetically-modified-foods.aspx.

-"Here's the Smarter Oil Alternative I Recommend to Replace Those Other Oils in Your Kitchen." Dr. Joseph Mercola's website. http://products.mercola.com/coconut-oil/

-"Juicing: Your Key to Radiant Health." Dr. Joseph Mercola's website. http://juicing.mercola.com/sites/juicing/juicing.aspx.

-"Learn the Truth About Soy: Just How Much Soy Do Asians Eat?" Dr. Joseph Mercola's website. January 9, 2000. http://articles.mercola.com/ sites/articles/archive/2000/01/09/truth-about-soy.aspx.

-"More Scientific Support for Using Olive Oil." Dr. Joseph Mercola's website. http://articles.mercola.com/sites/articles/archive/2005/01/29/olive-oil-part-three.aspx.

-"The Negative Health Effects of Chlorine." Retrieved from http://orthomolecular.org/library/jom/2000/articles/2000-v15n02-p089.shtml

-"Slathering on Sunscreen Does Not Prevent Cancer." Dr. Joseph Mercola's website. http://articles.mercola.com/sites/articles/archive/2003/08/02/sunscreen-cancer.aspx.

-"Tap Water Toxins: Is Your Water Trying to Kill You?" Dr. Joseph Mercola's website. February 7, 2009. http://articles.mercola.com/sites/articles/archive/2001/01/07/chlorinated-water2.aspx.

-"Vitamin B12: Are You Getting It?" Dr. Mercola's website. January 30, 2002. www.mercola.com/2002/jan/30/vitamin_b12.htm.

National Institutes of Health website. February 17, 2009. nccam.nih.gov/health/probiotics/D345.pdf.

National Review of Medicine, June 15, 2007. http://www.nationalreviewofmedicine.com/issue/2007/06_15/4_patients_practice04_11.html.

Natural Health School website. www.naturalhealthschool.com/acid-alkaline.html.

"Natural Secret to Heal Most Health Problems Revealed to US Public." *Vegetarian Times*, February 2001.

Nature.org website. www.nature.org/ourinitiatives/urgentissues/ rainforests/rainforests-facts.xml.

Navratilova, Martina. "Eat the Right Kinds of Protein: Don't Overdo Protein; Do it Right. Here's How." *AARP*, May 22, 2009.

Nazor, Nina. "All About Insulin." People and Diabetes website. peopleanddiabetes.com/id26.html.

Nielsen, Forrest. "Do You Have Trouble Sleeping? More Magnesium Might Help." USDA's Agricultural Research Service website. www.ars.usda.gov/News/docs.htm?docid=15617&pf=1&cg_id=0.

"Not Such Sweet News About Agave." *Berkeley Wellness Alert*, December 17, 2010. www.berkeleywellnessalerts.com/alerts/healthy_eating/ Agave-Versus-Refined-Sugar211-1.html.

"Nutrition of Sprouting Seeds." Livestrong website. www.livestrong.com/article/288551-nutrition-of-sprouting-seeds/#ixzz1AZqr74pP.

O'Connor, Anahad. "The Claim: Cinnamon Oil Kills Bacteria." New York Times, September 7, 2009. www.nytimes.com/2009/09/08/health/08real.html.

Office of Dietary Supplements of the US Government website. nccam.nih.gov/health/supplements/wiseuse.htm.

Ogden, Lillie. "The Environmental Impact of a Meat-Based Diet." *Vegetarian Times*, February 2001. www.vegetariantimes.com/ features/ft_eco_living/574.

O'Neil, John. "Vital Signs: Nutrition; Cooking Broccoli, Out of the Box." *The New York Times*. October 21, 2003. http://www.nytimes.com/2003/10/21/health/vital-signs-nutrition-cooking-broccoli-out-of-the-box.html.

Ott, John. *Light, Radiation and You: How to Stay Healthy*. Devin-Adair Publishers, 1982.

Pearson, Owen. "Vegetarian Foods Containing the B-5 Vitamin." Livestrong website. www.livestrong.com/article/339181-vegetarian- foods-containing-the-b-5-vitamin/#ixzz1SYBEgBD2.

Pereira, M.A. and V.L., Fulgoni, 3rd. "Consumption of 100% Fruit Juice and Risk of Obesity and Matabolic Syndrome: Findings from the National Health and Nutrition Examination Survey 1999–2004." *Journal of the American College of Nutrition*. 29(6), December 2010:625–9.

"Phytoestrogens and Breast Cancer—Fact Sheet #01." Revised July 2001. Cornell University website. envirocancer.cornell.edu/fact-sheet/diet/ fs1.phyto.cfm.

Pitchford, Paul. *Healing With Whole Foods*. North Atlantic Books, 2002.

Plourde, CLS,NCMP, PhD, Elizabeth. "Exposing the Hazards of Sunscreen." *Price-Pottenger Journal* Vol. 36, No. 1.

Pollack, Dr. "Water: The Single Most Important Element for Your Health." January 29, 2011. Dr. Mercola newsletter. http://articles.mercola.com/sites/articles/archive/2011/01/29/dr-pollack-on-structured-water.aspx.

Popke, Michael. "Studies Reveal More Chlorine Risks, Including Cancer." Athletic Business website. September 14, 2010. athletic-business.com/editors/blog/default.aspx?id=236.

Pottenger, Francis Marion. *Pottenger's Cats: A Study in Nutrition by Francis Marion Pottenger*. Price-Pottenger Nutrition Foundation, June 1, 1995.

"Probiotic Identified to Treat Ulcers (Counters H. pylori)." American Society for Microbiology. February 24, 2011. Free Republic website. www.freerepublic.com/focus/f-chat/2679352/posts.

"Professionals Urge End to Water Fluoridation." NewsLI website. November 25, 2007. www.newsli.com/2007/11/25/professionals-urge-end-to-water-fluoridation/.

Raloff, Janet. "Vitamin D Boosts Calcium Potency." Science News website. www.sciencenews.org/view/generic/id/6775/title/Food_for_Thought_Vitamin_D_Boosts_Calcium_Potency.

Regan, Tom. *The Case for Animal Rights*. University of California Press, 1983.

Robbins, John. "Diet for a New America." Veg Source website. www.vegsource.com/news/2009/09/how-to-win-an-argument-with-a-meat-eater.html.

- "2,500 Gallons All Wet?" Earthsave website. www.earthsave.org/environment/water.htm.

Rose, Natalia. *The Raw Food Diet Detox*. HarperCollins Publishers, 2006.

Rutz, Jim. "The Trouble with Soy." WorldNetDaily website. 2010. www.wnd.com/news/article.asp?ARTICLE_ID=53327.

Sandy Simmons's Connective Tissue Disorder website. www.ctds.info/index.html.

Schlosser, Eric. Fast Food Nation: *The Dark Side of the American Meal.* HarperCollins, 2002.

"School Drinking Water Unsafe: Schools in All 50 States, Especially Those with Private Supplies, Contain High Levels of Toxins." CBSNews— Healthwatch website. September 25, 2009. www.cbsnews.com/ stories/2009/09/25/health/main5338720.shtml?-source=related_ story

Sheegan, Daniel M., and Daniel R. Doerge. Letter to Dockets Management Branch (HFA-305). February 18, 1999. The letter was posted on the abcnews.com website as "Scientists Protest Soy Approval."

Shomon, Mary. "The Controversy over Soy and Thyroid Health." About.com website. May 27, 2009. thyroid.about.com/cs/soyinfo/a/soy_3. htm.

Simontacchi, C. *The Crazy Makers: How the Food Industry Is Destroying Our Brains and Harming Our Children*. Penguin, 2008.

Singer, Peter. *Practical Ethics*. Cambridge University Press, 1999.

Sircus, Dr. Mark. "Diabetes—Acid Conditions and Treatment with Sodium Bicarbonate." New Paradigms of Diabetic Care website. http://diabetic.imva.info/index.php/treatments/diabetes-acid-conditions-and-treatment-with-sodium-bicarbonate/.

"The Secrets of Light: Cancer and the Sun." Nourished Magazine website, December 2008. nourishedmagazine.com.au/blog/articles/the-secrets-of-light-cancer-and-the-sun.

Smith, Derek. "What Are the Benefits of Calcium Bentonite Clay?" Livestrong website. www.livestrong.com/article/201565-what-are-the-benefits-of-calcium-bentonite-clay/#ixzz1N7bf1183.

Staciokas, Linden. "Growing Sprouts Is Easy, Nutritious Way to Satisfy Veggie Cravings." *Fairbanks Daily News-Miner*, April 20, 2010. www.newsminer.com/view/full_story/7148528/article-Growing-sprouts-is-easy--nutritious-way-to-satisfy-veggie-cravings-.

Sterling, Joseph. "Secrets of Robust Health" newsletter. Healing Waters website. www.healingwatersforhealth.com/GetAttachment.pdf.

"Stevia." Tufts University Medical Center website. www.tuftsmedicalcenter.org/apps/Healthgate/Article.aspx?chunkiid=21876.

Stillwell, Sophie. "Vegetarian Sources of B Vitamins." Livestrong website. www.livestrong.com/article/208601-vegetarian-sources-of-b-vitamins/#ixzz1SYDIiRlw.

"Summary of NRDC's Test Results: Bottled Water Contaminants Found." Natural Resources Defense Council website. www.nrdc.org/water/drinking/bw/appa/asp.

"Sunscreens Exposed: 9 Surprising Truths. EWG's Skin Deep—Sunscreens 2011." Environmental Working Group website. June 23, 2011. http://www.ewg.org/enviroblog/2011/06/9-surprising-truths-about-sunscreen/.

Tabak, Alan J. "Magnesium-Rich Foods Reduce Diabetes Risk, Study Says." *Harvard Crimson*, January 21, 2004.

Tuntipopipat, Siriporn, Kunchit Judprasong, Christophe Zedet, Emorn Wasantwisut, Pattanee Winichagoon, Somsri Charoenkiatkul, Richard Hurrell, and Thomas Walczyk. "Chili, but Not Turmeric, Inhibits Iron Absorption in Young Women from an Iron-Fortified Composite Meal." *The Journal of Nutrition, Volume 136*, 2006: 2970–2974.

Tandel, Kirtida R. "Sugar substitutes: Health controversy over perceived benefits." US National Library of Medicine, *J Pharmacol Pharmacother*. 2011 Oct-Dec; 2(4): 236–243. doi: 10.4103/0976-500X.85936. PMCID: PMC3198517.

U.S. Department of Health and Human Services, National Toxicology Program. NTP TR 478. "NTP technical report on the toxicology and carcinogenesis studies of diethanolamine." Case no. 111-42-2. 1997.

Walsh, RD, Stephen. "Vegan Society B12 Factsheet." Vegan Society website. www.vegansociety.com/lifestyle/nutrition/b12.aspx.

Weigel, Jen. "Healthy Eating with a Spiritual Twist." Chicago Now website. July 20, 2009. www.chicagonow.com/blogs/spiritual-dammit/2009/07/healthy-eating-with-a-spiritual-twist.html#ixzz1S8wMYSoL.

Weil, Dr. Andrew website. www.drweil.com.

"What We Eat in America, NHANES 2001–2002, 1 Day, Individuals 1+ Years, Excluding Breast-Fed Children and Pregnant or Lactating Females." Agricultural Research Service website. www.ars.usda.gov/ SP2UserFiles/Place/12355000/pdf/0102/usualintaketables2001-02.pdf.

"Where Exactly Does Vitamin B12 Come From?" The Vegan Forum website. www.veganforum.com/forums/archive/index.php/t-6856.ht.

White, Scott. "The Benefits of Glutamine Supplements." Article 2008 website. article2008.com/Art/60332/561/The-Benefits-of-Glutamine-Supplements.html.

Wigmore, Ann and the Hippocrates Health Institute, Inc. *The Wheatgrass Book: How to Grow and Use Wheatgrass to Maximize Your Health and Vitality*. Avery Health Guides, 1985.

Wilens, T.E., J. Biederman, T.J. Spencer, J. Frazier, J. Prince, J. Bostic, M. Rater, J. Soriano, M. Hatch, M. Sienna, RB Millstein, and A. Abrantes. "Controlled Trial of High Doses of Pemoline for Adults with Attention-Deficit/Hyperactivity Disorder." *Journal of Clinical Psychopharmacology*, June 1999, 19(3):257–64.

Wilson, Dr. Lawrence. "Vitamin D Update 2010." Dr. Lawrence Wilson's website. www.drlwilson.com/ARTICLES/VITAMIN%20D.htm.

Yerba Prima website. www.yerba prima.com.

Young, PhD, Robert O., and Shelley Redford. *The Ph Miracle for Weight Loss*. New York and Boston: Warner Wellness, 2006.

Young Living Oils (brochure). "Rub A Dub Dub...Is Cancer In Your Tub?" Network News and Publications, 1999.

Endnotes

[1] "A different kind of school lunch." Pure Facts. October 2002. http://www.feingold.org/PF/wisconsin1.html.

[2] "Red Dye 40: Could It Cause Kids to Be Hyper?" http://www.wltx.com/story/news/2014/02/11/1673602/

[3] Marvin Boris, MD, and Francine S. Mandel, PhD. "Food and Additives are Common Causes of the Attention Deficit Disorder in Children." Annals of Allergy. October 1994, Volume 73 , October 1994.

[4] Dr. Joseph Mercola. "First Ever Study Reveals Amounts of Food Dyes in Brand Name Foods." May 22, 2014. Newsletter. http://articles.mercola.com/sites/articles/archive/2014/05/22/artificial-fooddyes. aspx.

[5] Ibid.

[6] Sarah Kobylewski, Ph.D. Candidate. Food Dyes: A Rainbow of Risks. Center for Science in the Public Interest. Molecular Toxicology Program. University of California. p. vi.

[7] Ibid. p. 15.

[8] Bruce H. Lipton, PhD. "Happy Healthy Child: A Holistic Approach." An Interview with Bruce Lipton by Sarah Kamrath. February 7, 2012. https://www.brucelipton.com/resource/article/happy-healthy-child-holistic-approach

[9] Jenny Hope. "Why a whiff of rosemary DOES help you remember: Sniffing the herb can increase memory by 75%." The Daily Mail. April 8, 2013. http://www.dailymail.co.uk/health/article-2306078/Why-whiff-rosemary-does-helpremember. html#ixzz3IOMsUxpt.

[10] Bruce H. Lipton, PhD. "Are You Programmed at Birth?" http://www.healyourlife.com/are-you-programmed-at-birth

[11] "Doing it on Your Own: Eating Vegetarian." McGill University website. June 30, 2010. www.mcgill.ca/fitatmcgill/nutrition/doingit/veg/.

[12] www.nutrientrich.com/1/prevent-and-reverse-heart-disease.html.

[13] John McDougall, MD. "Nutrition in the Medical Clinic Part III" lecture."Plant-Based Nutrition." Cornell University.

[14] T. Colin Campbell. "Principles of Nutritional Health" and "Plant-Based Nutrition." Cornell University and the T. Colin Campbell Foundation. 2010.

[15] Ibid.

[16] Yokoyama, Y., Barnard, N.D., Levin, S.M., Watanabe, M. Vegetarian diets and glycemic control in diabetes: a systematic review and meta-analysis. Cardiovasc Diagn Ther 2014. 4:373–382.

[17] Ibid.

[18] Ibid.

[19] Rachel Hennessey. "GMO Food Debate In The National Spotlight." Forbes 11/03/2014. http://www.forbes.com/sites/rachelhennessey/2012/11/03/gmo-food-debate-in-the-national-spotlight/2/

[20] Ibid.

[21] Joël Spiroux de Vendômois et al. "A Comparison of the Effects of Three GM Corn Varieties on Mammalian Health." Research paper. Int J Biol Sci 2009; 5(7):706-726. doi:10.7150/ijbs.5.706.

[22] Sanches, Albert et al. "Role of sugars in human neutrophilic phagocytosis." American Journal of Clinical Nutrition: http://ajcn.nutrition.org/content/26/11/1180.abstract#fn-1.

[23] Dr. Pollack. "Water: The Single Most Important Element for Your Health." January 29, 2011. Dr. Mercola newsletter. http://articles.mercola.com/sites/articles/archive/2011/01/29/dr-pollack-on-structured-water.aspx

[24] Ibid.

[25] Gabriel Cousens, MD. There Is A Cure For Diabetes. North Atlantic Books, Berkeley, Calif. 2008. p. 47.

[26] "Probiotic Identified to Treat Ulcers." Science News website. February 24, 2011. www.sciencedaily.com/releases/2011/02/110224121905.htm.

[27] "An Introduction to Probiotics." National Institutes of Health website. February 17, 2009. http://nccam.nih.gov/health/probiotics.

[28] "Expert Pediatrician Exposes Vaccine Myths" at http://articles.mercola.

com/sites/articles/archive/2009/11/14/expert-pediatrician-exposes-vaccine-myths.aspx

[29] From the question and answer library on Dr. Andrew Weil's website. Published December 11, 2002; updated March 21, 2005. www.drweil.com/drw/u/id/QAA142995.

[30] American Journal of Clinical Nutrition 50, 1997, p. 1264.

[31] Dr. Gregory Damato. "GM-Soy: Destroy the Earth and Humans for Profit." Natural News website. May 27, 2009. http://www.naturalnews.com/026334_soy_Roundup_GMO.html.

[32] Fallon, Sallon, and Mary G. Enig, PhD. "Soy's Dark Side: Newest Research on Why You Should Avoid Soy." DC Nutrition website. www.dcnutrition.com/news/Detail.CFM?RecordNumber=480.

[33] Ibid.

[34] Dr. Gregory Damato. "GM-Soy: Destroy the Earth and Humans for Profit." Natural News website. May 27, 2009. www.naturalnews.com/026334_soy_Roundup_GMO.html#ixzz1RzIZAWwh.

[35] Dr. Joseph Mercola. "Learn the Truth About Soy: Just How Much Soy Do Asians Eat?" Dr. Mercola's website. January 9, 2000. http://articles.mercola.com/sites/articles/archive/2000/01/09/truth-about-soy.aspx#!

[36] Fallon, Sallon, and Mary G. Enig, PhD. "Soy's Dark Side: Newest Research on Why You Should Avoid Soy." DC Nutrition website. www.dcnutrition.com/news/Detail.CFM?RecordNumber=480.

[37] Andy Bellatti. "You Ask, I Answer: Soy Protein Isolate." Medpedia.com website. April 16, 2011. http://smallbites.andybellatti.com/you-ask-i-answer-soy-protein-isolate/

[38] Daniel M. Sheegan, and Daniel R. Doerge. Letter to Dockets Management Branch (HFA-305). February 18, 1999. The letter was posted on the abcnews.com website as "Scientists Protest Soy Approval."

[39] Jim Rutz. "The Trouble with Soy." World Net Daily website. www.wnd.com/news/article.asp?ARTICLE_ID=53327. 2010. This article was originally titled "Soy Is Making Kids 'Gay'," but after a huge backlash he re-titled it "The Trouble with Soy."

[40] Andy Bellatti. "You Ask, I Answer: Soy Protein Isolate." Medpedia.com website. April 16, 2011. http://smallbites.andybellatti.com/you-ask-i-answer-soy-protein-isolate/

[41] Dr. David Brownstein. Salt Your Way To Health, 2nd edition. Medical Alternative Press. 2012. p. 17.

[42] Ibid. p. 26.

[43] Ibid. p. 53

[44] "Reduction in Blood Pressure with a Low Sodium, High Potassium, High Magnesium Salt in Older Subjects with Mild to Moderate Hypertension," British Medical Journal 301: 436–40, www.bmj.com/content/309/6952/436.

[45] Frances Sheridan Goulart. "Are you sugar smart?" American Fitness. March 1, 1991. http://www.highbeam.com/doc/1G1-10722552.html

[46] https://www.osha.gov/pls/oshaweb/owadisp.show_document?p_table=standards&p_id=10078.

[47] Ibid.

[48] Michael Edwards. "Healthy Sugar Alternatives: Understanding Both Healthy & Not So Healthy Sugars with Their Glycemic Index." Organic Lifestyle, June 12. 2009. http://www.organiclifestylemagazine.com/healthysugar- alternatives/ (This is a good source for the glycemic index of various sugars.)

[49] US National Library of Medicine, J Pharmacol Pharmacother. 2011 Oct-Dec; 2(4): 236–243. Kirtida R. Tandel. "Sugar substitutes: Health controversy over perceived benefits." http://www.ncbi.nlm.nih.gov/pmc/articles/PMC3198517/.

[50] "Methanol Poisoning." http://www.nlm.nih.gov/medlineplus/ency/article/002680.htm.

[51] Mark Gold. "Recall Aspartame as a Neurotoxic Drug." http://www.fda.gov/ohrms/dockets/dailys/03/jan03/012203/02p-0317_emc-000199.txt. nationalreviewofmedicine.com/issue/2007/06_15/4_patients_practice04_11.html

[52] Michael Edwards. "Healthy Sugar Alternatives: Understanding Both Healthy & Not So Healthy Sugars with Their Glycemic Index." Organic Lifestyle, June 12. 2009. http://www.organiclifestylemagazine.com/healthysugar- alternatives/ (This is a good source for the glycemic index of various sugars.)
[53] Mission Possible 1994, Stoddard 1995.
[54] The information from this section comes from Fran Gare's The Sweet Miracle of Xylitol. Basic Health Publications, Inc., 2003.
[55] "Cinnamon and Honey." Weekly World News. January 17, 1995.
[56] Gittleman, PhD, CNS, Ann Louise. Get the Sugar Out. Three Rivers Press, 1996. p. 15.
[57] The Importance of Breastfeeding, Office of the Surgeon General (US); Centers for Disease Control and Prevention (US); Office on Women's Health (US). Rockville (MD): Office of the Surgeon General (US); 2011. http://www.ncbi.nlm.nih.gov/books/NBK52687/
[58] Ibid.
[59] National Review of Medicine, June 15, 2007. http://www.
[60] National Review of Medicine, June 15, 2007. http://www.nationalreviewofmedicine.com/issue/2007/06_15/4_patients_practice04_11.html.
[61] Ibid.
[62] Albert Sanchez, J. L. Reeser, H. S. Lau, P. Y. Yahiku, R. E. Willard, P. J. McMillan, S. Y. Cho, A. R. Magie, and U. D. Register. "Role of sugars in human neutrophilic phagocytosis." The American Society for Clinical Nutrition, Inc. 1973. http://ajcn.nutrition.org/content/26/11/1180.abstract
[63] University of California. Berkeley Wellness Report. "Two Preservatives to Avoid." February 01, 2011. http://www.berkeleywellness.com/healthy-eating/food-safety/article/two-preservatives-avoid
[64] Healthy Eating Index, USDA, United States Department of Agriculture. http://www.cnpp.usda.gov/sites/default/files/healthy_eating_index/HEI99-00report.pdf.

[65] http://www.fitness.gov/eat-healthy/why-is-it-important/

[66] Study suggests nutrient decline in garden crops over past 50 years, Dec. 1, 2004, University of Texas: http://www.utexas.edu/news/2004/12/01/nr_chemistry/ For more information contact Lee Clippard, College of Natural Sciences, 512-232-0675.

[67] Ibid.

[68] Bryan Cohen. "Natural Cures for Enlarged Thyroid." eHow website. www.ehow.com/way_5317305_naturalcures- enlarged-thyroid.html#ixzz1SYtyAarn.

[69] Dr. David Brownstein, M.D. Iodine, Why You Need It; Why You Can't Live Without It. 4th edition. Medical Alternatives Press. 2009. pp. 228–229.

[70] "What We Eat in America, NHANES 2001–2002, 1 day, Individuals 1+ Years, Excluding Breast-Fed Children and Pregnant or Lactating Females." The US Department of Agriculture, Agricultural Research Service website. September 2005. www.ars.usda.gov/SP2UserFiles/Place/12355000/pdf/0102/usualintaketables2001-02.pdf.

[71] Ciarallo L, Brousseau D, Reinert S. "Higher-dose intravenous magnesium therapy for children with moderate to severe acute asthma."Arch Pediatr Adolesc Med. 2000;154(10):979.

[72] Forrest Nielsen. "Trouble Sleeping? More Magnesium Might Help." The US Department of Agriculture, Agricultural Research Service website. www.ars.usda.gov/News/docs.htm?docid=15617&pf=1&cg_id=0.

[73] Ibid.

[74] National Institutes of Health, Office of Dietary Supplements, Chromium, Dietary Supplement Fact Sheet. http://ods.od.nih.gov/factsheets/Chromium-HealthProfessional/#h10.

[75] Hendler SS, Rorvik D, eds. "PDR for Nutritional Supplements." Medical Economics. Montvale (NJ), 2001.

[76] Shils ME, Olson JA, Shike M. Modern Nutrition in Health and Disease, 9th ed. Williams & Wilkins, Balt., 1999.

[77] R. Thiel. "Natural vitamins may be superior to synthetic ones." Med Hypo, 2000;55(6):461-469.

[78] Dr. Joseph Mercola. "Slathering on Sunscreen Does Not Prevent Cancer." Dr. Joseph Mercola's website. articles.mercola.com/sites/articles/archive/2003/08/02/sunscreen-cancer.aspx.

[79] Dr. John Douillard, DC. "Vitamin D Has Astonishing Health Benefits." Dr. John Douillard's Lifespa.com website. http://www.lifespa.com/vitamin-d-has-astonishing-health-benefits/.

[80] Dr. John Douillard, DC. "Sun Exposure: Don't Be Fooled By Your Sunscreen." Dr. John Douillard's http://lifespa.com/dont-be-fooled-by-your-sunscreen/

[81] Dr. John Douillard, DC. "Vitamin D Has Astonishing Health Benefits."Dr. John Douillard's Lifespa.com website. http://www.lifespa.com/vitamin-d-has-astonishing-health-benefits/

[82] Ibid.

[83] "Exposing the Hazards of Sunscreen." Elizabeth Plourde, CLS,NCMP, PhD. Price-Pottenger Journal Vol. 36, No. 1.

[84] "Sunscreens Exposed: 9 Surprising Truths. EWG's Skin Deep—Sunscreens 2011." Environmental Working Group website. June 20, 2011. http://www.ewg.org/enviroblog/2011/06/9-surprising-truths-about-sunscreen/.

[85] Linus Pauling Institute for Micronutrient Research for Optimum health. OSU- Oregon Stare Universityhttp://lpi.oregonstate.edu/infocenter/lifestages/children/#RDA_4_to_8_yr –.

[86] James W. Anderson, Belinda M. Smith, and Nancy J. Gustafson. "Health benefits and practical aspects of high-fiber diets1'2," American Society for Clinical Nutrition .1994. 59(suppl):1242S-7S.

[87] S. Ji. "Wheat Contains Not One, but 23K Potentially Harmful Proteins." http://www.greenmedinfo.com/blog/wheat-contains-not-one-23k-potentiallyharmful- proteins.

[88] Jeffrey M. Smith. "Can Genetically Engineered Foods Explain the Exploding Gluten Sensitivity?" Institute for Responsible Technology Research. www.GlutenandGMOs.com

[89] Ibid.

[90] Joseph G. Hattersley. "The Negative Health Effects of Chlorine." Retrieved from http://orthomolecular.org/library/jom/2000/articles/2000-v15n02-p089.shtml

[91] Michael, Popke. "Studies Reveal More Chlorine Risks, Including Cancer." Athletic Business website. September 14, 2010. http://www.athleticbusiness.com/studies-reveal-more-chlorine-risks-including-cancer.html.

[92] Paul Connett, PhD. "50 Reasons to Oppose Fluoridation." St. Lawrence University (Canton, N.Y.). These "50 Reasons" were first compiled by Paul Connett and presented in person to the Fluoridation Forum in Ireland in October 2000. The document was refined in 2004 and published in Medical Veritas. See: http://fluoridealert.org/articles/50-reasons/ (It explained that after over four years the Irish authorities had not been able to muster a response to the "50 Reasons," despite agreeing to do so in 2000.)

[93] Ibid.

[94] Revisting the Fluoride-Osteosarcoma connection in the context of Elise Bassin's findings: Part 1 by Dr. Paul Connett, Chris Neurath and Michael Connett, submitted to the NRC review on the Toxicology of Fluoride in Water- page 1. March 2, 2005.

[95] Ibid.

[96] JV Kumar and Green, EL. Recommendations for Fluoride Use in Children, NY State Dental Journal, February, 1998. 41-48. Source: 50 Reasons to Oppose Fluoridation by Dr. Paul Connett, Professor of Chemistry, St. Lawrence University, 315-229-5853, eevideo@northnet.org.Human Services, National Toxicology Program. NTP TR 478. Two year study concluded 1997.

[97] Paul Connett, PhD. "50 Reasons to Oppose Fluoridation." St. Lawrence University. Canton, NY. These "50 Reasons" were first compiled by Paul Connett and presented to the Fluoridation Forum in Ireland in 2000. The document was refined in 2004 and published in Medical Veritas. www.fluoridealert.org/50reasons.htm.

[98] Levine, 1976, Ferjerskov, Thylstrup and Larsen, 1981; Carlos, 1983, Featherstone, 1987, 1999, 2000, Margolis and Moreno, 1990, Clark, 1993; Burt, 1994; Shellis and Duckworth, 1994 and Limeback, 1999, 2000), and the Centers for Disease Control and Prevention. (CDC, 1999).

[99] Paul Connett, PhD. "50 Reasons to Oppose Fluoridation." St. Lawrence University. Canton, NY.

[100] P. Galletti, Joyet, G. Effect on Flourine on Thyroidal Iodine Metabolism in Hyperthyroidism. Journal of Clinical Endocrinology. 1958. 18:1102-1110. http://www.fluoridealert.org/galletti.htm.

[101] Ditkoff, Lo Gerfo, P. The Thyroid Guide. Harper-Collins. 2000.

[102] F. F. Lin et al. The relationship of a low–iodine and high–fluoride environment to subclinical cretinism in Xinjiang. Iodine Deficiency Disorder Newsletter 7. 1991.

[103] Toxicological Profile for fluorides, Hydrogen /fluoride and Fluorine (F), US Department of Health and Human Services, ATSDR/ TP-91/17.1993.

[104] R.N. Hoover, R. N. et al. Fluoridation of Drinking Water and Subsequent Cancer Incidence and Mortality. Report to the Director of the National Cancer Institute. 1990

[105] Revisting the Fluoride-Osteosarcoma connection in the context of Elise Bassin's findings: Part 1 by Dr. Paul Connett, Chris Neurath and Michael Connett, submitted to the NRC review on the Toxicology of Fluoride in Water- page 1. March 2, 2005.

[106] M. Diesendorf, M. The Mystery Of The Declining Dental Decay. Nature. 322, 125-129. 1986.

[107] J. Colquhoun. "Why I changed my mind on fluoridation." Perspectives in Biology and Medicine. 41, 29-44. 1997. http://www.fluoride-journal.com/98-31-2/312103.htm

[108] Eliza Barclay. "What's Best for Kids: Bottled Water or Fountains?" National Geographic Daily News. March 3, 1020. news.nationalgeographic.com/news/2010/02/100303-bottled-water-tap-schools/.

[109] Associated Press. "Drinking Water at Schools Contains Lead, Pesticides, Other Toxins: Study." New York Daily News. September 25, 2009. http://www.nydailynews.com/life-style/health/drinking-water-schools-lead-pesticides-toxins-study-article- 1.404089

[110] "Bottled Water: Pure Drink or Pure Hype?" Natural Resources Defense Council website. www.nrdc.org/water/drinking/bw/bwinx.asp.

[111] Dr. Joseph Mercola. "Juicing: Your Key to Radiant Health." Dr. Mercola's website. http://articles.mercola.com/sites/articles/archive/2011/11/13/benefits-of-juicing.aspx.

[112] Ann Wigmore and Hippocrates Health Institute, Inc. The Wheatgrass Book: How to Grow and Use Wheatgrass to Maximize Your Health and Vitality. Avery Health Guides, 1985.

[113] Dr. Bernard Jensen. Health Magic Through Chlorophyll from Living Plant Life. Jensen's Health and Nutrition, 1973.

[114] Nina Nazor. "All About Insulin." People and Diabetes website. peopleanddiabetes.com/id26.html.

[115] Dr. Joseph Mercola. "Juicing: Your Key to Radiant Health." Dr. Mercola's website. http://articles.mercola.com/sites/articles/archive/2011/11/13/benefits-of-juicing.aspx.

[116] Diana Dyer, MS, RD. "What's in Kale? USDA Nutrient Content Data." 365 Days of Kale weblog. February 22, 2009. www.365daysofkale.com/2009/02/whats-in-kale-usda-nutrient-content.html.

[117] Jim Bolen. "Histamine/Anti-histamine and the Dangers of TakingAnti-histamine." Water Cure website. www.watercure2.org/histamines.htm.

[118] Fereydoon, Batmanghelidj, MD, ABC of Asthma, Allergies and Lupus, First Edition. Global Health Solutions, Inc., 2000.

[119] Paul Pitchford. Healing with Whole Foods, Third Edition. North Atlantic Books, 2002. pp. 224–5.

[120] Ibid., p. 537.

[121] Ibid., p. 545.

[122] Ibid., p. 246.

[123] PLB143: Evolution of Crop Plants. P. Gepts The crop of the day, Phoenix dactylifera. http://www.plantsciences.ucdavis.edu/GEPTS/pb143/CROP/DATE/date.htm.

[124] Science Daily, Raisins as a Functional Food for Oral Health. June 13, 2005. http://www.sciencedaily.com/releases/2005/06/050613062724.htm.

[125] "Amazing Benefits of Sleeping on Your Left Side." John Douillard, June 27, 2013. http://lifespa.com/amazing-benefits-of-sleeping-on-your-left-side.

[126] Anahad O'Connor. "The Claim: Cinnamon Oil Kills Bacteria." New York Times. September 7, 2009. http://www.nytimes.com/2009/09/08/health/08real.html?_r=0.

[127] "Ntp technical report on the toxicology and carcinogenesis studies of diethanolamine." (case no. 111-42-2) U.S. Department of Health and

[128] "Rub A Dub Dub...Is Cancer In Your Tub." Network News and Publications 1999. Young Living Oils brochure. https://www.youngliving.org/oils4wellness.

[129] Journal of the American Medical Association (JAMA) 3/15/95 Nutrition Health Review, Summer, 1995. n73, p.8 and U.S. News and World Report, March 17, 1997. v122 n10, p. 77.

[130] "High-Alcohol Mouthwashes Are Under Scrutiny." Oxford Journals Medicine & Health, JNCI J Natl Cancer Inst. Volume 83, Issue 11. pp. 751.

[131] Flavour and Fragrance Journal. 2008; 23. P. 444–449.

[132] Sue Chao, Gary Young, Craig Oberg, and Karen Nakaoka. "Inhibition of MRSA by essential oils." Young Living Essential Oils. Weber State University. January 2008.

[133] Ann Wigmore and Hippocrates Health Institute, Inc. The Wheatgrass Book: How to Grow and Use Wheatgrass to Maximize Your Health and Vitality. Avery Health Guides, 1985.

[134] "Honey and Cinnamon Cure." Weekly World News. January 17, 1995. http://weeklyworldnews.com/search/Honey+and+Cinnamon+Cure/.

[135] Dr. Joseph Mercola. "Everything You HAVE TO KNOW about Dangerous Genetically Modified Foods." Dr. Joseph Mercola's website. October 17, 2009. articles.mercola.com/sites/articles/archive/2009/10/17/everything-you-have-to-know-about-dangerousgenetically- modified-foods.aspx.

[136] Linden Staciokas. "Growing Sprouts Is Easy, Nutritious Way to Satisfy Veggie Cravings." Fairbanks Daily News-Miner. April 20, 2010. http://www.newsminer.com/features/food/growing-sprouts-is-easy-nutritious-way-to-satisfy-veggiecravings/article_fcdbf007-b718-5962-a8cb-d9904df23774.html.

[137] Sol Azulay. International Specialty Supply website. www.sproutnet.com/sprouts_in_the_press.htm.

[138] "Code of Federal Regulations, Title 21, Volume 2." Revised as of April 1, 2009. US Government Printing Office, GPO Access CITE: 21CFR101.22. pp. 72–76.

[139] Eric Schlosser. Fast Food Nation. Perennial, an imprint of Harper Collins, 2001- 2002. p. 126.

[140] Ibid.

[141] "Consumer Group Calls for Ban on 'Flour Improver': Potassium Bromate Termed a Cancer Threat." Center for Science in the Public Interest website. July 19, 1999. www.cspinet.org/new/bromate.html.
[142] Ibid.
[143] Rory Freedman and Kim Barnouin. Skinny Bitch. Running Press, 2005. p. 58.
[141] "Consumer Group Calls for Ban on 'Flour Improver': Potassium Bromate Termed a Cancer Threat." Center for Science in the Public Interest website. July 19, 1999. www.cspinet.org/new/bromate.html.
[142] Ibid.
[143] Rory Freedman and Kim Barnouin. Skinny Bitch. Running Press, 2005. p. 58.
[144] Dr. Stephen Wangen. "Milk Allergies and Lactose Intolerance." Food Allergy Solutions Review. News, Ideas & Strategies to Improve Your Health. July 2003. http://www.foodallergysolutions.com/food-allergy-news0307.html
[145] Rory Freedman and Kim Barnouin. Skinny Bitch. Running Press, 2005. p. 59.
[146] Theodore Gray. "A Change to Heat-Resistant Glass Has Had explosive Effects." PopSci website. April 26, 2011. www.popsci.com/science/article/2011-03/gray-matter-cant-take-heat.
[147] John McDougall, MD. "Alzheimer's Again Linked to Aluminum." Rense.com website. www.rense.comgeneral137/alum.htm.
[148] Amanda Schaffer. "Nervous About Nonstick? Easy to Clean and Incredibly Popular, This Cookware Is Still Considered Potentially Toxic by Some Experts. Good Housekeeping Settles the Debate—and Tells You How to Use it Safely." Good Housekeeping website. http://www.goodhousekeeping.com/product-reviews/cooking-tools/cookware-reviews/nonstick-cookwaresafety- facts
[149] Ibid.

[150] "Effects of microwave radiation on anti-infective factors in human milk." Quan R1, Yang C, Rubinstein S, Lewiston NJ, Sunshine P, Stevenson DK, Kerner JA Jr. Pediatrics. 1992. Apr;89(4 Pt 1):667-9.http://www.ncbi.nlm.nih.gov/pubmed/1557249

[151] John O'Neil. "Vital Signs: Nutrition; Cooking Broccoli, Out of the Box." The New York Times. October 21, 2003. http://www.nytimes.com/2003/10/21/health/
vital-signs-nutrition-cooking-broccoli-out-of-thebox. html.

[152] Betty Kamen, PhD, and Michael Rosenbaum, MD. "Microwaved Veggies: Bad News." Journal of the Science of Food and Agriculture 2003; 93(14), October 2003.

[153] Emily Main. "This or That: Bleach vs. Vinegar to Kill Germs." Rodale News. http://www.rodalenews.com/natural-disinfectant

Made in the USA
San Bernardino, CA
21 February 2015